FOOD AND BEVERAGE CONSUMPTION AND HEALTH SERIES

THE SALMONELLA OUTBREAK IN PEANUT PRODUCTS: THE FDA VS. GREED

FOOD AND BEVERAGE CONSUMPTION AND HEALTH SERIES

Additional books in this series can be found on Nova's website under the Series tab.

Additional E-books in this series can be found on Nova's website under the E-book tab.

FOOD AND BEVERAGE CONSUMPTION AND HEALTH SERIES

THE SALMONELLA OUTBREAK IN PEANUT PRODUCTS: THE FDA VS. GREED

BENJAMIN K. GLYNN
EDITOR

Nova Science Publishers, Inc.
New York

For permission to use material from this book please contact us:
Telephone 631-231-7269; Fax 631-231-8175
Web Site: http://www.novapublishers.com

LIBRARY OF CONGRESS CATALOGING-IN-PUBLICATION DATA

The salmonella outbreak in peanut products : the FDA vs. greed / editor, Benjamin K. Glynn.
p. ; cm.
Includes bibliographical references and index.
ISBN 978-1-60741-950-1 (hardcover : alk. paper)
1. Salmonella food poisoning--United States. 2. Peanuts. 3. United States. Food and Drug Administration. I. Glynn, Benjamin K.
[DNLM: 1. United States. Food and Drug Administration. 2. Salmonella Food Poisoning--etiology--United States. 3. Arachis hypogaea--United States. 4. Disease Outbreaks--prevention & control--United States. 5. Food Contamination--legislation & jurisprudence--United States. 6. Food Inspection--legislation & jurisprudence--United States. 7. Food Inspection--standards--United States. WC 268 S172 2009]
RA644.S15S235 2009
615.9'529344--dc22

2009031975

Published by Nova Science Publishers, Inc. † New York

CONTENTS

PREFACE

This book looks at the latest outbreak of Salmonella Typhimirum which started in September 2008. The illnesses peaked in December 2008, affecting consumers in 43 states. Though the illnesses have declined since the first announcement on January 10, 2009 that the suspected cause was peanut butter, they have not abated. The Salmonella strain has been linked to contaminated products from Peanut Corporation of America. As of January 29, 2009, there have been eight deaths and 550 illnesses linked to PCA's products. Thus this book also examines the PCA outbreak, which like countless episodes in the previous decade, illustrates numerous failures and areas where improvements are needed. This is an edited, excerpted and augmented edition of various government publications.

In: The Salmonella Outbreak in Peanut Products: The FDA … ISBN: 978-1-60741-950-1
Editor: Benjamin K. Glynn

Chapter 1

FAILURE TO PROTECT FOOD SUPPLY HEARING- COWART TESTIMONY

Darlene M. Cowart

Mr. Chairman my name is Darlene Cowart; you have my biographical information in the record. My education has been in biology and food science. I have worked in the agricultural commodity and food related quality control area since completing my education. I am currently President of JLA, USA. Our company is one of several under the umbrella of JLA Global which has facilities in the U.S. and overseas. JLA, USA has testing facilities in seven locations in the United States. While the majority of our work is related to the peanut industry we also provide services and testing to the almond industry and to some degree other food businesses. JLA, USA maintains microbiology laboratories in Albany, Georgia and Edenton, North Carolina.

We provide a broad range of testing services to the agricultural commodity and food business.

I understand the committee's concerns today relate to the recent salmonella outbreak and therefore involve our microbiology testing.

MICROBIOLOGY TESTING PROCEEDURES

Mr. Chairman when we test for salmonella we receive from the customer samples of the product to be tested together with a notification of the tests the customers wants us to perform. Specifically, we receive a "Request for Analysis," which details the battery of tests desired by the customer and includes the customer's description of the product to be tested. You have copies of these documents in the record.

I have also furnished the committee staff a detailed description of the method we use to test for Salmonella. I will simply summarize that method here.

First we pull a representative sample from the customer's containers to get a 375 gram composite sample. We put that composite sample with other substances into a sterile bag and incubate the mixture. We move some of the mixture into test tubes for other procedures and we put the remaining mixture into what is called a VIDAS machine. The machine's computer automatically gives the result—either positive or negative for Salmonella.

If the result is negative then we issue a negative certificate of analysis (COA) which is sent to the customer.

If the result is positive, we call that a presumptive positive which must be confirmed because, at this point several organisms can look like Salmonella but are not. However, since the tests necessary to confirm the presumptive positive can take five (5) days, we notify the customer of the presumptive positive by email and telephone call.

The confirmation process is quite technical and is described in the paper we furnished the committee staff.

If, after the confirmation process, we find that Salmonella is ruled out we prepare a negative COA for immediate release to the customer. If we do confirm the presumptive positive to be Salmonella then we prepare and issue a positive COA and again notify the customer via telephone call and email.

Mr. Chairman all these procedures conform to appropriate FDA and accepted laboratory standards.

PEANUT CORPORATION OF AMERICA SAMPLES

From January 1, 2007 through September of 2008 we tested approximately 1,000 samples of product for PCA. Of these in 2007 six (6) samples were confirmed positive for salmonella and all the rest were negative. In 2008 we issued a total of four (4) confirmed salmonella positive COA's.

I wish to emphasize, Mr. Chairman, that we at JLA do not take the samples from the product nor do we have knowledge of the sampling procedure used by PCA for the samples we receive

With respect to PCA samples, on each occasion that JLA received samples, the product samples would have been sent by mail to a JLA laboratory together with a Request for Analysis. The information provided on the Request for Analysis is the only information about the sample that JLA receives.

Following a confirmed salmonella positive issued to PCA in late August 2008, PCA discontinued sending product samples to JLA with one exception. JLA did receive and test a few samples sent under the name "PP Sales". It is my understanding that this name is an internal designation within PCA and refers to a different product line. JLA did test and obtain a confirmed salmonella positive on a PP Sales sample sent to JLA in late September 2008. A positive COA was issued to PCA in early October 2008.

In every instance when we found presumptive positives or confirmed positives we reported the results to PCA by email and telephone as I described earlier.

SALMONELLA GENERALLY

Salmonella can occur in raw agricultural commodities. The accepted procedure for killing salmonella in raw agricultural products is to heat the product to the necessary temperature for the appropriate period of time. That procedure is commonly referred to as a "kill step".

It is possible for Salmonella to be reintroduced into a product after the kill step. This can occur if the product comes into contact with contaminated raw ingredients, equipment or personnel. Therefore, it is extremely important that all food manufacturing facilities maintain appropriate procedures and processes to assure that recontamination does not occur.

Salmonella in processed food is preventable. The application of an appropriate kill step combined with manufacturing processes that eliminate the possibility of recontamination should result in a salmonella free product. Microbiological testing for salmonella, and other pathogens, is an important evaluative tool that manufacturers can, and should, employ to ensure that their manufacturing processes are safe.

Mr. Chairman we are cooperating fully with the committee and your staff. JLA pledges to continue working with the committee to make certain the food supply is safe for all consumers.

Thank you Mr. Chairman.

DARLENE M. COWART

Darlene M. Cowart, Ph.D., is President of JLA USA headquartered in Albany, Georgia. She has been employed by JLA USA for 9 years. Prior to joining JLA USA, Darlene was Food Safety Coordinator and Quality Assurance Manager for Cargill Peanut Products. Her primary responsibility was the implementation and management of the food safety and quality systems for a peanut butter plant, a peanut crushing plant, and three peanut shelling facilities. Darlene was employed by Cargill for five years. Darlene received a Bachelor's degree in Biology from Presbyterian College (1989), a Master's Degree in Horticulture from the University of Georgia (1991), and a Ph.D. in Food Science from the University of Georgia (1993).

In: The Salmonella Outbreak in Peanut Products: The FDA … ISBN: 978-1-60741-950-1
Editor: Benjamin K. Glynn

Chapter 2

FAILURE TO PROTECT FOOD SUPPLY HEARING-DEIBEL TESTIMONY

Charles T. Deibel

Good morning Chairman Stupak and members of the Subcommittee. I would like to thank you for giving me the opportunity to speak to you today. My name is Charles Deibel and I am president of Deibel Laboratories, Inc., a firm that specializes in micro-testing food and personal care products and food safety consulting.

BACKGROUND OF DEIBEL LABORATORIES, INC.

We have ten laboratories in North America, with headquarters in Illinois. For more than forty years, Deibel Labs has provided scientific consulting services to food manufacturers around the country. My father, who remains active in the company today, started the Deibel Labs when he was dean of the University of Wisconsin's bacteriology program in the late 1960's. He is widely recognized as one of the most knowledgeable scientists in the food industry, pioneering testing methods still in use today and helping to shape many food safety systems.

Deibel Labs is a member of numerous industry and professional organizations, including the International Association for Food Protection. Deibel Labs' professionals also are members of such organizations, including the Institute of Food Technologists, the International Association of Food Processors, the National Restaurant Association, and the National Confectionary Association. Many of our professionals are also certified as GMA-Safe and NFPA-Auditors and conduct training in numerous food safety programs.

In addition to micro-testing food products and their ingredients, we work with many manufacturers to help evaluate their existing food safety systems, conduct risk assessments, perform plant audits, and offer training in food safety procedures.

Dealings with Peanut Corporation of America and Cooperation With the Ongoing Investigations of the Peanut-Related Salmonella Outbreak

I want to give you a brief summary of Deibel Labs' dealings with Peanut Corporation of America or "PCA." My company did not provide day-to-day testing services for PCA as we do for many of our clients. Most relevant here, during 2007 and 2008, PCA's Plainview, Texas and Blakely, Georgia facilities sporadically submitted samples containing peanuts to Deibel Labs to test.

We have voluntarily cooperated with the Centers for Disease Control ("CDC"), the Food and Drug Administration ("FDA") and this Subcommittee to provide detailed records of the exact nature and timing of the tests that we performed for PCA's facilities, including samples from PCA's Blakely facility that tested "positive" for Salmonella in late September 2008 and the records of our immediate communications of those results to PCA's Blakely facility personnel. We also provided records detailing the requests that personnel at the Blakely facility made to us to re-test existing samples and the "negative" results of those tests.

It is not unusual for Deibel Labs or other food testing laboratories to find that samples clients submit do test positive for Salmonella and other pathogens, nor is it unusual that clients request that samples be re-tested. What is virtually unheard of is for an entity to disregard those results and place potentially contaminated products into the stream of commerce.

Considerations Impacting the National Food Safety System

I commend this Subcommittee for examining what can be done to prevent an incident like this from occurring again. As discussions progress on how to best to reform our national food safety system, I urge you to look at the entire model used today.

Our nation's current food safety system relies heavily on inspections conducted by the FDA and the state agencies with which it contracts. This is a reactive response, rather than the comprehensive, systemic process needed to safeguard our food. We believe that the FDA should focus on quality-control systems that minimize the potential for contamination to occur in the first place and develop mitigating strategies that correct a potential issue before it impacts food safety.

The FDA has a great deal of knowledge and understanding of how manufacturers can improve food safety practices. Our nation's small and medium sized companies, in particular, could greatly benefit from guidance documents from FDA. Yet, the FDA's job is to inspect, not to provide guidance, and so they do not do so. Yet, the United States Department of Agriculture ("USDA") routinely issues guidance documents to the food processors under its jurisdiction. FDA staff is reluctant to point manufacturers to the information and resources they need, or provide direct guidance on how an observation can be corrected. As a result, opportunities to improve food production practices are missed.

Testing, like inspection, is only one piece of an overall food safety policy. It is the last chance to catch a problem. The larger piece is on the front end–quality-control systems that minimize the potential for contamination to occur in the first place.

Every year, millions of pounds of food products end up in landfills because of positive tests for harmful organisms. The problem is not in a finding a positive result for such organisms from a test of a sample of its product—the issue we are discussing here is that a firm having commissioned testing of its product that found a positive, apparently attempted to test that same product into compliancy, and then released the product to the public anyway.

This attention to the issue of food safety is an opportunity to build stronger bridges between the FDA and food manufacturers. By taking a preventative, systemic approach, we can implement reforms that will go a long way towards ensuring that all consumers have access to a safe and wholesome food supply.

Thank You.

In: The Salmonella Outbreak in Peanut Products: The FDA … ISBN: 978-1-60741-950-1
Editor: Benjamin K. Glynn

Chapter 3

FAILURE TO PROTECT FOOD SUPPLY HEARING-HURLEY (FATHER) TESTIMONY

Peter K. Hurley

February 11, 2009

To:
United States House of Representatives
Committee on Energy and Commerce
Subcommittee on Oversight and Investigations

From:
Peter K. Hurley and family
Wilsonville, Oregon

RE:
Salmonella poisoning of Jacob M. Hurley due to his eating contaminated peanut butter crackers from a Peanut Corporation of America processed product.

My name is Peter Hurley. My wife Brandy and I are the parents of three children; Lauren 5 years old, Jacob 3 years old and Alyssa 8 months old. I am a police officer in Portland, Oregon and my wife is a marketing manager for a car dealership.

Our whole family, baby and all, have traveled from Oregon to Washington, D.C. to testify before you regarding the salmonella outbreak that has affected us, as well as hundreds and if not more likely thousands of fellow Americans.

I want to take a moment to acknowledge the eight the families who have lost a loved one. Eight people have died due to PCA's willful negligence. We were just lucky. It could have been very different for us.

We made this journey to appear before you because we felt it important enough for you to hear our story of how the Peanut Corporation of America (PCA) poisoned our son. We want you to hear how Jacob and a PCA supplied product are genetically linked in hopes that you will take action to protect our food supply; so that Americans do not have to worry about even the simplest of foods killing their loved ones.

Jacob's story began with him becoming ill with diarrhea and vomiting in early January 2009. He appeared to be coming down with the flu. He was sallow, lethargic and probably had a fever that we did not catch. In a few days he began to have blood in his diarrhea. Knowing that blood in the stool is serious and needs immediate attention, we took him to the pediatrician who sent us home with a fecal collection kit. A few days later the pediatrician called to let us know that the lab results had come back and that Jacob had salmonella poisoning! He stated that we should expect a phone call from our county health department.

At this point we did not know how Jacob got the poisoning and because of that we did not know how to protect the rest of the family. All we knew was the Jacob had Salmonella poisoning and that five or six people had all ready died in a new outbreak linked to peanut butter. But, at the time only KING NUT PEANUT BUTTER was listed as a source, which we knew we did not have. We called Jacob's school to see if other children were sick, and none were. At that point we began to feel helpless in not knowing what got him sick. What had we unknowingly given him that gave him salmonella poisoning?

As Jacob's diarrhea continued, my wife was given the OK from our pediatrician's office for Jacob to eat his favorite comfort food, AUSTIN TOASTY CRACKERS WITH PEANUT BUTTER!! The very food that we later found was the cause of his poisoning! So, here we have a boy who is trying to get over food poisoning and one of the foods that would seem safe even, to people in the pediatric medical community, is the exact product that is continuing to poison him.

A week after we received the initial results of salmonella poisoning from the doctor, we spoke with a staff member of the State of Oregon's Office of Disease Prevention and Epidemiology. By this time there was initial information coming out that peanut products were looking like the link to a nation wide salmonella outbreak. The next day the epidemiologist for the Sate of Oregon, Dr. William Keene, came to our house, himself, at five o'clock on a Saturday night. As a friend said this is like having the head of the FBI coming out to take fingerprints. I have to commend Dr. Keene on his dedication to make such a visit. On that Saturday night Dr. Keene took custody of our supply of AUSTIN TOASTY CRACKERS WITH PEANUT BUTTER, manufactured by KELLOGS, with PCA product in it.

One week later Dr. Keene called us to say that Jacob and the crackers he took from our house had an exact DNA-subtype match for Salmonella Typhimurium. Three out of six packages of crackers tested positive. ***This was the food that even the pediatrician thought safe enough for us to continue to feed him while he was sick!*** The issue was no longer what had we done unknowingly, but what had PCA done knowingly?

Jacob continued to have diarrhea for eleven days. Alyssa, our baby, was seven months old at the time. We had to be extremely vigilant with cleaning to ensure that there was never any cross contamination between Jacob and Alyssa. If Alyssa had come down with salmonella poisoning there is a good chance that we would be one of the families who lost a loved one due to PCA's willful negligence. We know from the FDA's most recent report that it was truly willful negligence.

I am using the word poisoned carefully here. I realize what I am saying. I have read the Food and Drug Administration's (FDA) most recent Form 483 report, dated 01/09/2009-

02/05/2009, regarding the plant where the peanut butter product for these crackers came from. This was not an accident. PCA knowingly allowed for tainted product to leave the plant, as well as allow it to stay in the production supply chain. It sickens me to no end that the majority of a company and its employees could knowingly allow tainted product to go out the door and into the nations food supply. Does no one have a conscience? Were people jut hoping that no one would get sick or die? People would be in utter outrage if they heard of a police officer putting a loaded gun to someone's head, pulling the trigger, and in the horrific aftermath say "I was just hoping that the bullet in the chamber wouldn't fire." NO, NO, NO! Both of these scenarios are utterly unacceptable. One is real and the other is fictitious, but neither should be real in the United States.

Never in my wildest dreams would I have thought I would be sitting before a Congressional subcommittee representing millions of Americans, begging for you to take action against a rouge food production company. But, that is what I am doing today. We, the Hurley family from Wilsonville, Oregon, have been affected by PCA and on behalf of millions of Americans, we need you to take action.

We, the United States, **are** the first world. Have we fallen to second world status for food supply safety? I think if you ask Americans who pay attention to what is happening in the world they would answer "YES" to this question. It has gotten to the point where we have a food safety crisis in America.

As the woman taking care of our dog while we are gone said, *"Even my dog is not safe! What is this, China?!"*

Where do we go from here? Well, being in the law enforcement profession, I see many parallels between food safety monitoring and control to that of criminal law enforcement. We need to have a faster 9-1-1 oriented medical response to food contamination, in order to prevent further innocent victims. You can liken this to an active shooter type scenario. In that situation you have someone who is actively shooting and killing people at random; as in a school or mall. In those incidents, people are begging for the police to go in and stop the killer. Well here you have food bacteria randomly killing innocent people. And just as with a shooter, the faster you stop the spread of the bacteria and or product, the fewer victims there will be.

So what does that mean in the real world? It means having state epidemiologists like Oregon's own Dr. Keene who will come to your house on a weekend night to collect evidence. Just like a police officer would do in a rape case. Criminals and bacteria do not work a day job. They are attacking us 24/7 and that is why epidemiologists need the resources across the country to do the same kind of work Dr. Keene was able to do.

You also need the cop on the beat approach as well. You need FDA inspectors out there with the authority to stop production immediately when there is a problem. It is like the police officer stopping two people from arguing in public before it turns into a fight, then a brawl and then a riot.

The FDA needs the ability to criminally prosecute quickly and effectively when needed. If someone is convicted of a felony in the criminal justice system, they go to prison and are not allowed to vote. But, if you poison Americans via their food supply what are the consequences? You pay a fine and keep producing? Is this right? Is this what we as Americans want? I can say with certainty it is NOT!

I would like for all of us to think of the worst case scenario here, food borne terrorism. Oregon has the dubious distinction as being the first place for domestic terrorism. It was carried out by the Rajneeshees, in the 1980's. They were a fanatical religiously based criminal group that was in the Oregon high desert. In 1985 they poisoned Wasco County residents at a restaurant salad bar in the town of The Dalles. They sprayed the salad bar with Salmonella. Over one hundred residents fell ill. It would have been much worse if they had only gotten the concentration levels correct. This act of domestic terrorism was carried out successfully almost twenty five years ago by a small group of religious fanatics in rural Oregon. If they could pull it off, who else could?

None of us should be so naive as to think that Al-Qaeda could not easily taint our food supply very effectively. If, the very-well funded Al-Qaeda put its mind to it, I shudder to think of what could happen to this country when people do not know where to turn to find safe, uncontaminated, food. The panic, pandemonium and lawlessness would be horrific.

So, now is the time to take action to protect our food supply before another national out break occurs, whether it is greed or terrorist motivated.

I will leave you with my favorite quote by the 19th Century author, poet and philosopher Johann Wolfgang Goethe:

"*Few men have imagination enough for reality.*"

On behalf of all Americans, my whole family, Jake and I ask you to please have enough imagination to think of the worst case reality and to protect against it.

With this I conclude my testimony to the Congressional Subcommittee on Oversight and Investigations for Energy and Commerce.

Thank you.

Respectfully,
Peter K. Hurley
Wilsonville, OR 97070

In: The Salmonella Outbreak in Peanut Products: The FDA … ISBN: 978-1-60741-950-1
Editor: Benjamin K. Glynn

Chapter 4

FAILURE TO PROTECT FOOD SUPPLY HEARING-PARNELL EMAIL1

Stewart Parnell

From: Stewart Parnell
Sent: Monday, October 06, 2008 8:39 AM
To: 'Sammy Ughtsey'
Cc: 'David Voth'

Subject RE: Granule:

We need to discuss this ....the time lapse , beside: the cost is coding us huge $$$$$ and causing obviously a huge lapse in time from the time we pick up peanuts until the time we can invoice..,

We need to find out somehow what our competition (JIMBOS) is doing and at the very least mimic their policy …

We need to protect our self and the problem is that the tests absolutely give us no protection, just an indication at best …

Let's talk.
Stewart

From: Sammy Ughtsey
Sent Monday, September 29, 2008 12:40 PM
To: stew.parnetal 'David Voth'
Subject: Granules

We received Final Lab results from Deibel this morning and we have a Positive for Salmonella. Lot 8268 of Granules produced last Thursdily. We, produced 441 cases of this lot and we produced meal out of the same lot. Samples are going out today for retesting and we will have results on Thursday. Some of this products has been shipped. 280 cases of 'Medium Chop to Field brook and 40 cases of Meal to Keny Ingredients. These customers need to be Called and the product placed on HOLD until this can be cleared. All remaining product is on HOLD in the plant. We have not had any High micro numbers of any kind in Granules and we completely disassembled the line this weekend for cleaning.

In: The Salmonella Outbreak in Peanut Products: The FDA … ISBN: 978-1-60741-950-1
Editor: Benjamin K. Glynn

Chapter 5

FAILURE TO PROTECT FOOD SUPPLY HEARING-PARNELL EMAIL2

Stewart Parnell

From: Stewart Parnell
Sent: 01/19/2009
To: robertmeligan
Cc: barbara.wood
Bcc:
Subject: FW: truck to TX

Bob,

This truck was shipped from our Blakely, GA facility last week to our Texas plant, you can see below what was on this thick, we do not want to use it in production unless you feel it is okay, Jan verbally gave Sammy the okay but now GA USDA is putting a hold on everything else in the plant.

Obviously we are not shipping any peanut butter products affected by the recall but desperately at least need to turn the Raw Peanuts on our floor into money..we have other raw peanuts on our floor that we would like to do the same with..

Could you give us advice on the status of this material this is material that would be cooked / further processed by us in our Texas facility and tested afterwards as all of our products are...

Thanks,
Stewart

From: Joe Sams
Sent: Monday, January 19, 2009 9:23 AM
To stewart.pamel 'Jesus Garrochot'; 'Sammy Lightsey'
Subject: RE: truck to TX

Raw B1 Jumbo Runners (3 lots) 31,264 lbs
Raw B1 Med Runners (2 lots) 12,000 lbs

In: The Salmonella Outbreak in Peanut Products: The FDA … ISBN: 978-1-60741-950-1
Editor: Benjamin K. Glynn

Chapter 6

Failure to Protect Food Supply Hearing-Parnell Email3

Stewart Parnell

From: Lynchburg Office'
Sent: Monday, January 12, 2009 3:19 AM
To: Sammy.lightse mary.wilkerson joe-sams
sherry.davis 'Steve Hutto'; manuel.brubake
frank.hardric Jesus Garrochos 'Lisa Ochoa; blanca.pen
brandy.sem balde.cenice
cathy.mullins 'Melissa Jones'; marc.poirie
grey.adams rish AticBride; lynnette.su GBPame stewart.pamell stewart.ada
Subject: Salmonella Investigation

Dear all:

Late last week, public health officials in Minnesota, while looking around a nursing home kitchen for the source of a salmonella food-sickness case, found salmonella in an already opened tub of our peanut butter made in Blakely and sold by King Nut under their brand. We suspect the salmonella could have been introduced by cross- contamination after the tub was opened. We do not believe the salmonella came from our facility. As you probably know, we send hourly PB samples to an independent lab to test for salmonella during production of peanut butter, and we have never found any salmonella at all.

No salmonella has been found anywhere else in our products or in our plants, or in any unopened containers of our product. It was found ONLY in an already opened container. The investigating agencies, the Food and Drug Administration and the Centers for Disease Control and Prevention, have NOT said they believe there is salmonella in any of our other product. They also have NOT stated that they believe we were the source of the salmonella found in the partially-used tub.

However, it is their responsibility to investigate thoroughly, and they are doing that right now.

Despite these minimal facts, news agencies are looking for a news story where there currently isn't one.

Please everyone: Media have the power to turn this open container misunderstanding into a disaster for this company's good name if we handle this wrong. If you get calls from media outlets (newspaper, TV, radio, etc.,) DO NOT answer any questions, even though the urge is nearly irresistible. Here's what to do if the news media call and you answer:

1. Politely tell them that PCA is eager to answer their questions.
2. Do not give your name.
3. Inform them that Stewart Pamell or his designee will be the only point of contact, per PCA company policy.
4. Offer to fax them our official press release on the matter. This press release is attached to this email and is also available on our Website at www.peanutcorp.com.
5. Tell them that you would be happy to jot down their questions and they can be assured they will be FIRST to receive those answers from our single point of contact.

If possible, try to determine their deadline. When do they need these answers by? Please make good notes of their questions; we will use them to issue a MA document to answer all similar questions.

ALSO:

1. Never say no comment." There's no worse thing to say to the media, ever. We DO have comments. We just want them to be accurate and from a single source.
2. Please inform all subordinates and coworkers that no one is to answer any media questions about anything, but politely send questioners to the Corporate Office or Stewart Pamell directly.
3. Media DO NOT have the right to enter our facility, or even to be on our property, unless specifically permitted by Stewart Pamell. We must, however, be polite to them.
4. Government investigators DO have the right to enter our facility.
5. DO make notes of what you notice we are doing right and wrong to handle this issue. We may face a similar misunderstanding again in the future and we want to use these lessons next time. Please keep and share your notes with the Lynchburg Office in the coming days.
6. Don't worry. We are well positioned to deal with this event no matter what happens. The most important thing for you to know is that we don't expect any surprises; our testing and safety procedures allow us to have great confidence that the opened container in Minnesota was contaminated long after it left our plant That's all the government agencies have found after 3 days (so far) of examining our operations closely with 0-tips and magnifying glasses. PCA's products are well-tested and safe; we were not the cause of this food-sickness outbreak.

Thanks for your predictable professionalism in a challenging situation. I look forward to talking with all of you as soon as we have more information. Please email me (stewart panell) with any media phone numbers or email addresses and their questions I need to answer.

Stewart Parnell, Gloria, Grey, and
everyone in the Lynchburg Office.
/SA

In: The Salmonella Outbreak in Peanut Products: The FDA … ISBN: 978-1-60741-950-1
Editor: Benjamin K. Glynn

Chapter 7

FAILURE TO PROTECT FOOD SUPPLY HEARING-PRONTO LETTER TO WAXMAN

Henry A. Waxman

February 10, 2009
Hon. Henry A. Waxman, Chairman, Committee of Energy and Commerce
Hon. Bart Stupak, Chairman, Subcommittee on Oversight and Investigations
U.S. House of Representatives
2125 Rayburn House Office Building
Washington, D.C. 20515

Dear Sirs,

In response to questions presented to me by Michael Gordon, Deputy Chief Investigative Counsel for Committee on Energy and Commerce, I am enclosing my responses in attached document.

Sincerely,

Michelle Pronto

1. Please briefly describe your professional history and your current position and responsibilities at J. Leek Associates, Inc. (JLA)

   RJR NABISCO-AVOCA MERRY HILL, NC MAY 1981-SEPT 1991 LAB TECHNICIAN
   ANDRITZ, INC. GLENS FALLS, NY DEC 1991-DEC 2003 LAB TECHNICIAN
   CIBA SUFFOLK, VA MAY 2005-NOV 2006 SHIFT CHEMIST

JLA EDENTON, NC NOV 2006-PRESENT MANAGER OF MICROBIOLOGY LAB

I CURRENTLY MANAGE THE MICROBIOLOGY LABS IN EDENTON, NC AND ALBANY, GA. I ACT AS COORDINATOR FOR THE EDENTON LAB AND SUPPORT THE ALBANY LAB AS MANAGER

2. Did PCA ever discuss with JLA its food safety controls, such as the effectiveness of its method for killing pathogenic bacteria in the roasting process? Please describe any communications you are aware of between JLA and PCA on this topic.

   ON 1/25/08, MR. PARKER (JLA) AND I PARTICIPATED IN A CALL WITH DANNY KILGORE (PCA) REGARDING A POTENTIAL ROASTER VALIDATION PROTOCOL. MR. PARKER HAD SENT AN EMAIL TO MR. KILGORE ON 1/23/08 TO SET UP THE CALL. TO MY KNOWLEDGE, A ROASTER VALIDATION PROTOCOL WAS NEVER RECOMMENDED AND PCA DID NOT FOLLOW UP WITH ME ON THIS SUBJECT.

3. Do you have any knowledge of whether Peanut Corporation of America (PCA) ever sought multiple test results for the same product — e.g., sent samples to multiple labs simultaneously, sought re-testing at the same or a different lab after receiving a test result, etc. If so, please provide all information you have about such instances, including whether JLA's initial results were confirmed upon re-testing. Please describe any communications you are aware of between JLA and PCA or internally within JLA on this topic.

   BASED UPON A REVIEW OF JLA RECORDS, IT APPEARS THAT PCA RE-SUBMITTED SAMPLES FOR TESTS OF COLIFORMS AND SALMONELLA. I DO NOT KNOW WHETHER THE SAMPLES WERE FROM THE SAME PRODUCT LOT BUT, IN JULY 2007, THREE DIFFERENT SAMPLES WITH A DESCRIPTION "7190B" WERE SUBMITTED AND TWO SAMPLES WITH A DESCRIPTION "7192A" WERE SUBMITTED FOR SALMONELLA. THE SAMPLES DESCRIBED AS 7190B CONFIRMED POSITIVE IN TWO TESTS, BUT TESTED NEGATIVE FOR SALMONELLA ON THE THIRD TEST. THE SAMPLES DESCRIBED AS "7192A" CONFIRMED POSITIVE IN ONE TEST AND NEGATIVE IN THE SECOND.

   ADDITIONALLY, DURING A PHONE CONVERSATION IN AUGUST 2008, SAMMY LIGHTSEY (PCA) INFORMED ME THAT THE ALBANY, GEORGIA JLA LAB WAS REPORTING HIGHER AEROBIC PLATE COUNT (APC) RESULTS AND HIGHER COLIFORM RESULTS THAN ANOTHER LAB HE HAD APPARENTLY USED. HE TOLD ME THAT HE HAD PULLED DUPLICATE SAMPLES SIMULTANEOUSLY AND SENT ONE SET OF SAMPLES TO JLA AND THE OTHER SET TO ANOTHER LAB, AND THAT OUR RESULTS WERE ALWAYS HIGHER FOR APC AND COLIFORM. I STATED THAT JLA FOLLOWS THE AOAC METHOD AND THAT I COULD NOT EXPLAIN THE DIFFERENCE. I TOLD HIM I WOULD REVIEW THE OTHER LAB'S RESULTS FOR COMPARISON. MR. LIGHTSEY SENT TWO REPORTS TO ME BY EMAIL ON 8/21/08 THAT WERE FROM ANOTHER LAB (DEIBEL). I COMPARED THE DATA TO THE JLA RESULTS. I MENTIONED MR. LIGHTSEY'S COMPLAINT IN AN EMAIL TO DARLENE COWART AND MIKE JACKSON DATED 9/12/08.

ADDITIONALLY, AFTER JLA ISSUED A CONFIRMED POSITIVE SALMONELLA TO PCA IN AUGUST 2008, MR. LIGHTSEY CALLED TO DISCUSS. A CONFERENCE CALL WAS SET UP WITH CERTAIN JLA EMPLOYEES AND PCA. MR. LIGHTSEY SAID HE HAD FLUSHED CERTAIN PIPES WITH HOT OIL. MR. LIGHTSEY WAS TOLD BY JLA THAT THIS MAY NOT BE SUFFICIENT TO KILL ANY SALMONELLA. DURING THIS CONFERENCE CALL, MR. LIGHTSEY REQUESTED THAT THE LAB INDIVIDUALLY TEST ADDITIONAL SAMPLES
FROM EACH OF THE SIX CUPS ORIGINALLY PROVIDED BY PCA. HE FURTHER TOLD ME HE WAS GOING TO SEND THE LAB ADDITIONAL SAMPLES TO TEST. I UNDERSTOOD THOSE TO BE HIS "RETAINED" SAMPLES. PCA DID NOT PROVIDE THOSE ADDITIONAL SAMPLES TO JLA FOR TESTING. JLA DID RUN ADDITIONAL TESTS FROM EACH OF THE 6 CUPS, AND OBTAINED NEGATIVE SALMONELLA RESULTS, WHICH WERE REPORTED TO PCA.

4. Do you have any other knowledge regarding whether PCA ever shipped products that had received a presumptive or confirmed positive test result for salmonella or other microbiological contamination? Please describe any communications you are aware of between JLA and PCA on this topic.

   I ONLY KNOW WHAT MR. LIGHTSEY SAID TO ME IN A CALL THAT TOOK PLACE IN EARLY OCTOBER 2008 AFTER A CONFIRMED SALMONELLA POSITIVE HAD APPARENTLY BEEN ISSUED BY JLA FOR A SAMPLE SENT UNDER THE NAME "PP SALES." WHEN I CALLED MR. LIGHTSEY IN EARLY OCTOBER 2008 TO GIVE HIM SEROLOGY RESULTS THAT JLA HAD OBTAINED FROM DEIBEL LAB FOR THE CONFIRMED SALMONELLA, HE PAUSED, SAID "UH OH," OR SOMETHING TO THAT EFFECT, AND THEN TOLD ME HE HAD RELEASED THE PRODUCT FOR SHIPPING. WHEN I ASKED IF HE COULD GET IT BACK, HE SAID IT WAS ON A TRUCK HEADED TO UTAH AND RATHER THAN GETTING IT BACK, HE WOULD HAVE THE PRODUCT DESTROYED SOMEWHERE OUT WEST. I DID NOT WRITE ANY NOTES ABOUT THE CONVERSATION, BUT I DID MENTION IT TO TWO JLA EMPLOYEES (MR. PARKER AND MR. JACKSON). I RECALL SAYING THAT MR. LIGHTSEY HAD ALREADY SHIPPPED PRODUCT AND THAT HE WAS GOING TO HAVE IT DESTROYED ON THE WEST COAST. MR. JACKSON MENTIONED THAT SHIPPING COSTS WERE HIGH AND THAT IT WOULD LIKELY BE LESS EXPENSIVE TO DESTROY THE PRODUCT OUT WEST.

5. Do you have any knowledge of whether PCA was dissatisfied or concerned about the salmonella, coliform, aerobic plate count, or other test results provided by JLA? Please describe any communications you are aware of between JLA and PCA on this topic.

   SEE RESPONSE TO QUESTION NUMBER THREE (3). ADDITIONALLY, MR. LIGHTSEY DID COMPLAIN ABOUT THE APC AND COLIFORM RESULTS. AS RELATED BELOW, SOMEONE AT PCA TOLD THE LAB COORDINATOR IN ALBANY (STEPHANIE FLETCHER) THAT PCA WAS NOT GOING TO SEND ADDITIONAL SAMPLES FOR TESTING TO JLA. THAT

CONVERSATION FOLLOWED MY DISCUSSION WITH MR. LIGHTSEY REGARDING HIS CONCERN WITH OUR LAB'S HIGH COLIFORM AND APC COUNTS.

6. Please describe any change you are aware of in the relationship between JLA and PCA in the last year. Specifically, did PCA reduce its use of JLA's testing services in the summer or fall of 2008? If so, why?
   I RECEIVED AN EMAIL ON 9/10/08 FROM JLA EMPLOYEE STEPHANIE FLETCHER STATING THAT SHE WAS TOLD BY THE QC MANAGER OF PCA THAT PCA WAS NO LONGER GOING TO SEND US SAMPLES, BUT THAT PP SALES GROUP WOULD CONTINUE TO SEND SAMPLES TO JLA. I CALLED MR. LIGHTSEY TO FOLLOW UP ON THE RECENT DISCUSSION REGARDING THE CONFIRMED POSITIVE, AND HE CONFIRMED THAT BECAUSE OF HIGH COLIFORM RESULTS THEY WERE GOING TO SEND SAMPLES TO A DIFFERENT LAB FOR AWHILE. WE DID NOT RECEIVE ANY SAMPLES LABELED "PCA" BETWEEN 8/26/08 AND 11/24/08. WE DID RECEIVE ONE PCA SAMPLE IN LATE NOVEMBER AND ISSUED A NEGATIVE SALMONELLA COA ON 12/1/08.
7. What knowledge do you have regarding how many times PCA's products tested positive for salmonella or other microbiological contamination? How does this compare to other clients of JLA?
   I DID NOT KNOW THIS INFORMATION, BUT HAVE SINCE REVIEWED DATA TO RESPOND TO THIS QUESTION. DATA IN OUR LIMS (LABORATORY INFORMATION MANAGEMENT SYSTEM) SHOWED THAT FROM 8/14/07, THE DATE WE BEGAN COLLECTING DATA IN LIMS, THROUGH 01/31/09 JLA TESTED APPROXIMATELY 1000 SAMPLES FOR PCA. OF THESE, 4 WERE POSITIVE FOR SALMONELLA. I HAVE NOT REVIEWED DATA FROM OTHER CLIENTS TO MAKE A COMPARISON.
8. Do you have any information about positive test results for salmonella in PCA products, the effectiveness of PCA's food safety controls, or microbiological contamination of PCA products that you have not already described? If so, please explain.
   I BELIEVE I HAVE ANSWERED THIS IN PREVIOUS QUESTIONS.
9. Please describe all communications you are aware of between JLA and PCA regarding an incident in which PCA product was contaminated with metal.
   I RECEIVED A PHONE CALL FROM MR. LIGHTSEY ON 6/27/08. HE STATED HE HAD PRODUCT STOPPED AT CANADIAN CUSTOMS WITH METAL CONTAMINATION. HE REQUESTED INFORMATION ON FEDERAL/STATE INSPECTION SERVICES. I TOOK HIS NUMBER AND PASSED IT AND A BRIEF DESCRIPTION OF PROBLEM ON TO DR. COWART. THAT'S THE EXTENT OF MY KNOWLEDGE ON THAT INCIDENT.
10. Have you had any communications with PCA since PCA's Blakely, GA plant was identified as a possible source of the current salmonella outbreak? If so, please describe all such communications.
    MR. LIGHTSEY CALLED ME ON 1/21/09. HE ASKED FOR REPORTS ON ANY SALMONELLA POSITIVES FOR PCA. HE FOLLOWED UP ON 1/22/09 TO SEE IF ALL SALMONELLA REPORTS HAD BEEN SENT. HE SAID THAT HE WAS

TRYING TO MATCH REPRINTS WITH OLD REPORTS. I ALSO CALLED MR. LIGHTSEY TO GET A RELEASE FROM PCA ALLOWING JLA TO HAVE DEIBEL LABS PROVIDE SLANTS TO FDA LIGHTSEY CALLED, READ THE RELEASE AND THEN EMAILED APPROVAL TO ME.

I EMAILED PCA TO GET THEIR PERMISSION TO RELEASE THEIR LAB REPORTS TO FDA ON 1/23/09.

MR. LIGHTSEY CALLED ON 1/24/09. HE ASKED IF JLA COULD SEND ALL REPORTS FROM 2007 AND 2008 TO HIM BY 3:35PM ON 1/25/09.

WE SENT AS MANY REPORTS AS WE COULD BUT COULD NOT MAKE DEADLINE. THERE WERE A COUPLE OF EMAILS PASSED ON 1/25 MAKING SURE THAT ALL REPORTS WERE BEING SENT TO THE CORRECT EMAIL ADDRESS AND THERE MAY HAVE BEEN A PHONE CALL. I TRIED TO CALL MR. LIGHTSEY TO TELL HIM WE COULD NOT MAKE DEADLINE, BUT DID NOT REACH HIM.

MR. LIGHTSEY CALLED ON 1/26/09 AND STATED HE STILL NEEDED THE REMAINING PAPERWORK BY 11:30AM ON 1/27/09. HE ALSO STATED THERE WAS A DISCREPANCY ON ONE OF THE COA'S REGARDING SAMPLE SIZE. ON 1/27/09, I SENT AN EMAIL SEEKING CLARIFICATION ON THE "DISCREPANCY'. MY EXAMINATION OF COA SHOWED NO DISCREPANCY, AND THE ISSUE WAS RESOLVED WITH MR. LIGHTSEY.

I HAD NO FURTHER CONTACT WITH PCA OR MR. LIGHTSEY.

In: The Salmonella Outbreak in Peanut Products: The FDA … ISBN: 978-1-60741-950-1
Editor: Benjamin K. Glynn

Chapter 8

FAILURE TO PROTECT FOOD SUPPLY HEARING-WAXMAN STATEMENT

Henry A. Waxman

Thank you, Chairman Stupak. I want to commend you on your leadership of this Subcommittee and thank you for calling today's hearing. I also want to commend Ranking Member Walden for his bipartisan work on this investigation.

For too long, the American people have not been able to trust that the food they eat is safe. From botulism in canned food to cattle that are too sick to even stand, our nation's food supply is at risk.

As we will hear during our first panel, those who most often pay the price are the young, elderly, and infirm. We know the tainted products distributed by the Peanut Corporation of America were sent to elementary schools, nursing homes, hospitals, and even FEMA meal kits handed out in the wake of the Kentucky ice storms.

Today the public will hear the first results of our investigation. The documents obtained by the Subcommittee are disturbing. They seem to show a company that was more concerned with its bottom line than the safety of its customers.

Last September, for example, PCA was notified by a private lab that its products had tested positive for salmonella. This wasn't the first positive test the company received, and it wouldn't be the last.

In response, the president of the company, Stewart Parnell, sent an email complaining that positive salmonella tests were "costing us huge $$$$$ and causing obviously a huge lapse in time from the time we pick up peanuts until the time we can invoice."

Even after FDA began investigating in January and forced the company to recall some products, PCA's first concern was financial.

On January 19, PCA's president, Mr. Parnell, sent an e-mail pleading with FDA officials to allow the company to keep doing business. He wrote that they "desperately at least need to turn the Raw Peanuts on our floor into money."

He assured FDA that these peanuts "would be cooked [and] further processed by us in our Texas facility." This is the same facility that was shut down yesterday after salmonella was found there too.

The Subcommittee has also obtained documents that appear to show that Mr. Parnell was not forthcoming about his company's past.

Despite multiple records showing positive salmonella tests over three years, Mr. Parnell wrote an e-mail to his company's employees on January 12, asserting flatly that "we have never found any salmonella at all."

He blamed "news agencies" that "are looking for a news story where there currently isn't one," and he declared that "we were not the cause of this food-sickness outbreak."

The Subcommittee also obtained a statement from an official at one of the private labs used by PCA to test for *salmonella.* The lab official reported that PCA's plant manager in Georgia, Sam Lightsey, admitted to shipping products before receiving lab results. The official stated:

> "When I called Mr. Lightsey in early October 2008 to give him the serology reports that JLA had obtained from Diebel lab for the confirmed salmonella, he paused, said "Uh Oh," or something to that effect, and then told me he had released the product for shipping. When I asked if he could get it back, he said it was on a truck heading to Utah."

This lab official also informed us that PCA stopped using its services because it received too many positive tests. The official stated:

> "I called Mr. Lightsey to follow up on the recent discussion regarding the confirmed positive, and he confirmed that because of the high coliform results they were going to send samples to a different lab."

Mr. Chairman, I ask that all of these documents be made part of the official hearing record.

During today's hearing, I hope we will be able to find out more about the actions of these PCA officials. I also look forward to hearing from the labs that conducted these tests, as well as the state and federal officials in charge of overseeing this company.

I also extend my deepest condolences to the victims and family members of victims who are here today.

In: The Salmonella Outbreak in Peanut Products: The FDA … ISBN: 978-1-60741-950-1
Editor: Benjamin K. Glynn

Chapter 9

FDA INSPECTION REPORT ON PEANUT CORP

Benjamin K. Glynn

DEPARTMENT OF HEALTH AND HUMAN SERVICES
FOOD AND DRUG ADMINISTRATION

DISTRICT ADDRESS AND PHONE NUMBER	DATE(S) OF INSPECTION
60 Eighth Street NE Atlanta, GA 30309 (404) 253-1161 Fax:(404) 253-1202 Industry Information: www.fda.gov/oc/industry	01/09/2009 - 02/05/2009* FEI NUMBER 1036857

NAME AND TITLE OF INDIVIDUAL TO WHOM REPORT ISSUED
TO: Sammy L. Lightsey, Plant Operations Manager

FIRM NAME	STREET ADDRESS
Peanut Corporation Of America	14075 Magnolia St
CITY, STATE, ZIP CODE, COUNTRY	TYPE ESTABLISHMENT INSPECTED
Blakely, GA 39823-1381	Peanut Roaster/Peanut Butter and Paste Manufacturer

This document lists observations made by the FDA representative(s) during the inspection of your facility. They are inspectional observations, and do not represent a final Agency determination regarding your compliance. If you have an objection regarding an observation, or have implemented, or plan to implement, corrective action in response to an observation, you may discuss the objection or action with the FDA representative(s) during the inspection or submit this information to FDA at the address above. If you have any questions, please contact FDA at the phone number and address above

DURING AN INSPECTION OF YOUR FIRM WE OBSERVED:

OBSERVATION 1

Failure to manufacture foods under conditions and controls necessary to minimize the potential for growth of microorganisms and contamination.

Specifically, the firm's private laboratory microbiological testing found the following:

Salmonella Typhimurium: Peanut paste under lot # 8278 was found contaminated with Salmonella Typhimurium by private laboratory testing conducted by the firm. After the firm retested the product and received a negative status, the firm shipped (b)(4) lb. of the product in interstate commerce. Additionally, this peanut paste was manufactured on 9/26/08 from (b)(4) lb. totes of roasted peanuts received on 9/25/08. The lots of roasted peanuts received on 9/25/08 were also used to produce the following products that were also shipped in interstate commerce: (b)(4) totes were used to manufacture (b)(4) peanut butter under lot # 8276, one tote was used to manufacture peanut butter for (b)(4) under lot # 8277 and (b)(4) (b)(4) under lot # 8277.

Creamy Stabilized Peanut Butter, manufactured on 8/11/08 (producing both lots #8220 and #8224), tested positive for Salmonella by (b)(4) received the PCA sample for these lots on 8/12/08 and issued a report of positive results on 8/27/08. The isolate from this sample was sent to (b)(4) and was confirmed as Salmonella Anatum. The firm then had this lot retested at both (b)(4) and (b)(4) with both labs finding negative results. However, PCA had already shipped into interstate commerce the following: An 8/15/08 shipment of (b)(4) lbs. (invoice #0107013) creamy stabilized peanut butter under lot #8220 went to (b)(4)

Lot #8268, Peanut Meal and Medium Chopped Peanuts, manufactured on 9/24/08, tested positive for Salmonella by (b)(4) (b)(4) received this PCA sample on 9/25/08 and issued a report of the positive results on 10/6/08. This sample was confirmed by (b)(4) as Salmonella Anatum. However, PCA had already shipped into interstate commerce the following lots before lab results were known: On 9/24/08 a shipment of (b)(4) lbs. (invoice #302583) of peanut meal under

AMENDED

	EMPLOYEE(S) SIGNATURE	DATE ISSUED
SEE REVERSE OF THIS PAGE	Janet B Gray, Investigator Darcy E. Brillhart, Microbiologist Sandra I. Gaul, Investigator Robert P. Neligan, Investigator Lesley K. Satterwhite, Microbiologist Theresa L. Stewart, Investigator	02/05/2009

FORM FDA 483 (9/08) PREVIOUS EDITION OBSOLETE INSPECTIONAL OBSERVATIONS PAGE 1 OF 5 PAGES

DEPARTMENT OF HEALTH AND HUMAN SERVICES
FOOD AND DRUG ADMINISTRATION

DISTRICT ADDRESS AND PHONE NUMBER	DATE(S) OF INSPECTION
60 Eighth Street NE Atlanta, GA 30309 (404) 253-1161 Fax:(404) 253-1202 Industry Information: www.fda.gov/oc/industry	01/09/2009 - 02/05/2009* FEI NUMBER 1036857

NAME AND TITLE OF INDIVIDUAL TO WHOM REPORT ISSUED
TO: Sammy E. Lightsey, Plant Operations Manager

FIRM NAME	STREET ADDRESS
Peanut Corporation Of America	14075 Magnolia St
CITY, STATE, ZIP CODE, COUNTRY	**TYPE ESTABLISHMENT INSPECTED**
Blakely, GA 39823-1891	Peanut Roaster/Peanut Butter and Paste Manufacturer

lot#8268 to (b)(4) On 9/25/08 a shipment of (b)(4) lbs. (invoice #1057536) medium chopped granules under lot #8268 went to (b)(4)

Lot #8168, Medium Chopped Peanuts and Peanut Meal, manufactured on 6/16/08 tested positive for Salmonella by (b)(4) (b)(4) received the PCA sample for this lot on 6/17/08 and issued a report with the positive results on 6/23/08. The firm resubmitted a sample to (b)(4) on 6/21/08 with a report issued on 6/23/08 as negative. This firm had shipped the following product into interstate commerce prior to receiving the sample results on 6/23/08: A shipment on 6/18/08 of (b)(4) lbs. (invoice #662837) of peanut meal under lot #8169 went to (b)(4) On 6/20/08 this firm shipped approximately (b)(4) lbs. (invoice #61108) of peanut meal under lot #8169 to (b)(4)

Lot #8161A, Small Chopped Peanuts, manufactured on 6/9/08, testing positive for Salmonella by (b)(4) (b)(4) received the PCA sample for this lot on 6/10/08 and issued a report with the positive results on 6/16/08. This firm resubmitted a sample to (b)(4) on 6/18/08 which was found to be negative per a report issued 6/21/08. PCA had already shipped product from lot# 8161A in interstate commerce before the positive results were known on 6/16/08. On 6/10/08 a shipment of approximately (b)(4) lbs. (invoice #MRB6408) of small chopped peanuts under lot #8161 went to (b)(4) On 6/13/08 a shipment of (b)(4) lbs. (invoice #11114-3) of small chopped peanuts under lot #8161 went to (b)(4)

Lot #8028, Peanut Paste, manufactured on 1/25/08 tested positive for Salmonella by (b)(4) received the PCA sample for this lot on 1/26/08. However, also on 1/26/08 PCA shipped (b)(4) lbs. (invoice #4503605302) of peanut paste under lot #8028 to (b)(4)

Salmonella (no strain identified): Medium Chopped Granules manufactured on January 24, 2008 under lot # 8024 tested positive for Salmonella by a private laboratory. After the firm retested the product and received a negative status, the product was shipped in interstate commerce.

Lot # 7206, Small Chopped Peanut Granules, manufactured on or around 7/26/07, tested positive for Salmonella by (b)(4) (b)(4) received the PCA sample on 7/26/07 and issued a report of the positive results on 7/30/07. PCA had already shipped approximately (b)(4) lbs (invoice #736434-001) of small chopped peanuts under lot #7206 to (b)(4) (b)(4) on 7/27/07 before the lab results were obtained.

Lot #7192A, Small Chopped Peanuts, manufactured on 7/11/07, tested positive for Salmonella by (b)(4) (b)(4) received the PCA sample for this lot on 7/12/07 and issued a report of the positive Salmonella results on 7/18/07. Two more samples of this lot were submitted to both (b)(4) and (b)(4) The (b)(4) follow-up sample of this lot submitted on 7/18/07 was classified negative on 7/19/07. The (b)(4) follow-up sample of this lot

AMENDED

	EMPLOYEE(S) SIGNATURE	DATE ISSUED
SEE REVERSE OF THIS PAGE	Janet B Gray, Investigator Darcy E. Brillhart, Microbiologist Sandra I. Gaul, Investigator Robert P. Neligan, Investigator Lesley K. Satterwhite, Microbiologist Theresa L. Stewart, Investigator	02/05/2009

FORM FDA 483 (04/03) PREVIOUS EDITION OBSOLETE **INSPECTIONAL OBSERVATIONS** PAGE 2 OF 8 PAGES

DEPARTMENT OF HEALTH AND HUMAN SERVICES
FOOD AND DRUG ADMINISTRATION

DISTRICT ADDRESS AND PHONE NUMBER	DATE(S) OF INSPECTION
60 Eighth Street NE Atlanta, GA 30309 (404) 253-1161 Fax:(404) 253-1202 Industry Information: www.fda.gov/oc/industry	01/09/2009 - 02/05/2009* FEI NUMBER 1036857

NAME AND TITLE OF INDIVIDUAL TO WHOM REPORT ISSUED
TO: Sammy L. Lightsey, Plant Operations Manager

FIRM NAME	STREET ADDRESS
Peanut Corporation Of America	14075 Magnolia St
CITY, STATE, ZIP CODE, COUNTRY	TYPE ESTABLISHMENT INSPECTED
Blakely, GA 39823-1881	Peanut Roaster/Peanut Butter and Paste Manufacturer

submitted on 7/18/07 was classified as positive for Salmonella.
Records show that PCA shipped product from this lot prior to receiving the analytical results on 7/18/07. On 7/12/07 a shipment of approximately (b)(4) lbs. (invoice #LALIT70507) of small chopped peanuts under lot #7192 went to (b)(4) (b)(4) Also, on 7/12/07 a shipment of (b)(4) lbs. (invoice #732153-001) of small chopped peanuts under lot #7192 went to (b)(4)

Lot #7190B, Medium Chopped Peanuts, manufactured on 7/9/07, tested positive for Salmonella by (b)(4) (b)(4) received two PCA samples for lot #7190B on 7/10/07 and 7/12/07. Both samples were positive with the lab reports issued on 7/16/07 and 7/18/07 respectively. The following shipments were released into interstate commerce before the final lab results were obtained: On 7/11/07 a (b)(4) lb. shipment of medium chopped peanuts (invoice #100986) under lot #7190 went to (b)(4) On 7/12/07 a (b)(4) lb shipment of medium chopped peanuts (invoice #18049-30) under lot #7190 went to (b)(4) On 7/13/07 a shipment of (b)(4) lbs of medium chopped peanuts (invoice #31810) under lot #7190 went to (b)(4) and on 7/13/07 a (b)(4) lb shipment of medium chopped peanuts (invoice #759) under lot #7190 went to (b)(4) Additionally, the firm made the following shipments on or after the positive Salmonella results were obtained: On 7/18/07 a shipment of (b)(4) lbs. of medium chopped peanuts (invoice #21479) under lot #7190 went to (b)(4) and on 7/24/07 a shipment of approximately (b)(4) lbs. of medium chopped peanuts (invoice #10872-2) under lot #7190 went to (b)(4) (b)(4)

Lot # 7190 B19-JR, Oil-Roasted Salted Jumbo Peanuts (b)(4) manufactured on 7/9/07 tested positive for Salmonella by (b)(4) received the PCA sample for this lot on 7/10/07 and issued a report of the positive results on 7/16/07. On 7/12/07 PCA submitted a second sample to (b)(4) of the same lot (#7190 B19-JR) and received a negative status for Salmonella on 7/16/07. The following shipments were released by PCA into interstate commerce before final lab results were known: A 7/10/07 shipment of (b)(4) lbs. (invoice #12131) oil roasted salted jumbo peanuts under lot #7190 went to (b)(4) A 7/12/07 shipment of (b)(4) lbs. (invoice #213157) oil roasted salted jumbo peanuts under lot #7190 went to (b)(4) A 7/12/07 shipment of approximately (b)(4) lbs. (invoice #213158) oil roasted salted jumbo peanuts under lot #7190 went to (b)(4) A 7/13/07 shipment of approximately (b)(4) lbs. (invoice #11463) oil roasted salted jumbo peanuts under lot #7190 went to (b)(4)

Lot # 7157, Small Chopped Peanut Granules, manufactured on 6/7/07, tested positive for Salmonella by (b)(4) (b)(4) received the PCA sample on 6/7/07 and issued a report of the positive results on 6/13/07. However, PCA had already shipped (b)(4) lbs (invoice # 721676-001) of small chopped peanuts under lot #7157 to (b)(4) (b)(4) on 6/7/07 before the lab results were obtained.

AMENDED

SEE REVERSE OF THIS PAGE	EMPLOYEE(S) SIGNATURE	DATE ISSUED
	Janet B Gray, Investigator Darcy E. Brillhart, Microbiologist Sandra I. Gaul, Investigator Robert P. Neligan, Investigator Lesley K. Satterwhite, Microbiologist Theresa L. Stewart, Investigator RPN	02/05/2009

FORM FDA 483 (04/03) PREVIOUS EDITION OBSOLETE INSPECTIONAL OBSERVATIONS PAGE 3 OF 8 PAGES

DEPARTMENT OF HEALTH AND HUMAN SERVICES
FOOD AND DRUG ADMINISTRATION

DISTRICT ADDRESS AND PHONE NUMBER	DATE(S) OF INSPECTION
60 Eighth Street NE Atlanta, GA 30309 (404) 253-1161 Fax:(404) 253-1202 Industry Information: www.fda.gov/oc/industry	01/09/2009 - 02/05/2009* FEI NUMBER 1036857

NAME AND TITLE OF INDIVIDUAL TO WHOM REPORT ISSUED

TO: Sammy L. Lightsey, Plant Operations Manager

FIRM NAME	STREET ADDRESS
Peanut Corporation Of America	14075 Magnolia St
CITY, STATE, ZIP CODE, COUNTRY	**TYPE ESTABLISHMENT INSPECTED**
Blakely, GA 39823-1881	Peanut Roaster/Peanut Butter and Paste Manufacturer

OBSERVATION 2

Failure to maintain equipment, containers and utensils used to convey, hold, and store food in a manner that protects against contamination.

Specifically, the peanut paste line was not cleaned after the Salmonella Typhimurium was isolated from the peanut paste manufactured on September 26. 2008 (lot # 8278). The firm continued to manufacture peanut paste in this system from 9/26/08 to the beginning of this inspection on 1/9/09. (b)(4) ots of peanut paste have been manufactured on this line between 9/26/08 and 1/9/09.

There are no records to document the cleaning of the peanut paste line after Salmonella was detected in peanut paste manufactured on January 25, 2008 (lot # 8028). The firm continued to manufacture peanut paste in this system.

AMENDED

	EMPLOYEE(S) SIGNATURE	DATE ISSUED
SEE REVERSE OF THIS PAGE	Janet B Gray, Investigator Darcy E. Brillhart, Microbiologist Sandra I. Gaul, Investigator Robert P. Neligan, Investigator Lesley K. Satterwhite, Microbiologist Theresa L. Stewart, Investigator	02/05/2009

FORM FDA 483 (04/03) PREVIOUS EDITION OBSOLETE INSPECTIONAL OBSERVATIONS PAGE 4 OF 8 PAGES

DEPARTMENT OF HEALTH AND HUMAN SERVICES
FOOD AND DRUG ADMINISTRATION

DISTRICT ADDRESS AND PHONE NUMBER	DATE(S) OF INSPECTION
60 Eighth Street NE Atlanta, GA 30303 (404) 253-1161 Fax:(404) 253-1202 Industry Information: www.fda.gov/oc/industry	01/09/2009 - 02/05/2009* FEI NUMBER 1036857

NAME AND TITLE OF INDIVIDUAL TO WHOM REPORT ISSUED
TO: Sammy L. Lightsey, Plant Operations Manager

FIRM NAME	STREET ADDRESS
Peanut Corporation Of America	14075 Magnolia St
CITY, STATE, ZIP CODE, COUNTRY	**TYPE ESTABLISHMENT INSPECTED**
Blakely, GA 39823-1681	Peanut Roaster/Peanut Butter and Paste Manufacturer

OBSERVATION 3

Failure to perform mechanical manufacturing steps so as to protect food against contamination.

Specifically, this firm recognizes the roasting step as the control point for eliminating microbiological contamination in raw materials. However, this firm has not established the effectiveness of the temperature, volume, or belt speed specific to this roaster to assure it is adequate as a kill step for pathogenic bacteria. Additionally, the firm's records of the roaster's temperature are inadequate in that dates have been left off of several circular recording charts. For example, in August 2008 three days of recording charts were not dated; in September 2008 two recording charts were not dated; in October 2008 six charts were not dated; in November 2008 24 days of recording charts were not dated; and in December 2008 and January 2009 no temperature recording charts were dated.

OBSERVATION 4

Failure to store finished food under conditions that would protect against microbial contamination.

Specifically, on 1/9/09 (b)(4) lb. totes of raw peanuts were observed to be stored directly next to (b)(4) lb. totes of finished, roasted peanuts in the firm's production/packaging room. The totes of finished product included the following: Honey Roasted Peanuts under lot # 8339; Dry Roasted Peanuts under lot # 9002; Peanut Meal under lot # 9005; and Dark Roasted Peanuts (paste line) under lot # 9009. The (b)(4) totes of raw peanuts were all under lot # 40147. On 1/26/09, an additional (b)(4) lb. tote of raw peanuts under lot # 16195-08 was observed to be stored in the production/packaging room along with the same lots of finished goods listed above. It was visually difficult to discern which of these totes were finished products and which were raw products.

The above totes of finished product were stored within 15 feet of a floor crack where an environmental swab was collected on 1/10/09 and found positive for Salmonella Senftenberg.

Also, one environmental swab collected on 1/10/09 from the finished product cooler floor (beside the south wall) was found positive for Salmonella Mbandaka. The swab location was within 3 feet of pallets of finished product.

Mold was observed growing on the ceiling and walls in the firm's cooler used for finished product storage. In addition, water stains were observed running down from the cooling unit fans in the cooler. On 1/10/09, pallets of finished product were stored directly beneath this unit.

AMENDED

	EMPLOYEE(S) SIGNATURE	DATE ISSUED
SEE REVERSE OF THIS PAGE	Janet B Gray, Investigator Darcy E. Brillhart, Microbiologist Sandra I. Gaul, Investigator Robert P. Neligan, Investigator Lesley K. Satterwhite, Microbiologist Theresa L. Stewart, Investigator	02/05/2009

FORM FDA 483 (04/03) PREVIOUS EDITION OBSOLETE INSPECTIONAL OBSERVATIONS PAGE 4 OF 8 PAGES

DEPARTMENT OF HEALTH AND HUMAN SERVICES
FOOD AND DRUG ADMINISTRATION

DISTRICT ADDRESS AND PHONE NUMBER	DATE(S) OF INSPECTION
60 Eighth Street NE Atlanta, GA 30309 (404) 253-1161 Fax:(404) 253-1202 Industry Information: www.fda.gov/oc/industry	01/09/2009 - 02/05/2009* FEI NUMBER 1036857

NAME AND TITLE OF INDIVIDUAL TO WHOM REPORT ISSUED
TO: Sammy L. Lightsey, Plant Operations Manager

FIRM NAME	STREET ADDRESS
Peanut Corporation Of America	14075 Magnolia St
CITY, STATE, ZIP CODE, COUNTRY	TYPE ESTABLISHMENT INSPECTED
Blakely, GA 39823-1081	Peanut Roaster/Peanut Butter and Paste Manufacturer

OBSERVATION 5

The plant is not constructed in such a manner as to allow ceilings to be kept in good repair.

Specifically, on 1/10/09 there were open gaps observed as large as 1/2" x 2 1/2 feet at the air conditioner intakes located in the roof of the firm. Water stains were also observed on the ceiling around the air conditioner intakes. Additionally, there were water stains and streaks located on the edges of the skylights where rain water has been leaking into the firm. All of these openings were located in the production/packaging room. Totes of finished, roasted product and a roasted nut packaging line are located directly underneath these areas.

OBSERVATION 6

The design of equipment and utensils fails to preclude the adulteration of food with contaminants.

Specifically, a felt material is present on the final roller at the roaster's discharge. This material cannot be adequately cleaned or sanitized.

Also, the rework kettle in the peanut butter room had openings (2" x 3") at the top exposing the peanut butter to open conditions.

OBSERVATION 7

Proper precautions to protect food and food-contact surfaces from contamination with microorganisms cannot be taken because of deficiencies in plant construction and design.

Specifically, the firm is not equipped with a ventilation system to prevent cross-contamination by providing a negative room pressure in the facility. A negative room pressure would direct air flow from the finished product areas into the negative pressure room (raw peanut receipt and staging area), ensuring that contaminated air does not escape to other parts of the facility.

The raw peanut receipt/staging area, peanut paste tanker line, peanut roasters, and the peanut granule line are housed in the same open room with no segregation. In addition, the honey roasted peanuts, considered to be finished product, are filled into

AMENDED

	EMPLOYEE(S) SIGNATURE	DATE ISSUED
SEE REVERSE OF THIS PAGE	Janet B Gray, Investigator Darcy E. Brillhart, Microbiologist Sandra I. Saul, Investigator Robert P. Neligan, Investigator RPN Lesley K. Satterwhite, Microbiologist Theresa L. Stewart, Investigator	02/05/2009

FORM FDA 483 (04/03) PREVIOUS EDITION OBSOLETE INSPECTIONAL OBSERVATIONS PAGE 6 OF 6 PAGES

DEPARTMENT OF HEALTH AND HUMAN SERVICES
FOOD AND DRUG ADMINISTRATION

DISTRICT ADDRESS AND PHONE NUMBER	DATE(S) OF INSPECTION
60 Eighth Street NE Atlanta, GA 30309 (404) 253-1161 Fax:(404) 253-1202 Industry Information: www.fda.gov/oc/industry	01/09/2009 - 02/05/2009* FEI NUMBER 1036857

NAME AND TITLE OF INDIVIDUAL TO WHOM REPORT ISSUED
TO: Sammy L. Lightsey, Plant Operations Manager

FIRM NAME	STREET ADDRESS
Peanut Corporation Of America	14075 Magnolia St
CITY, STATE, ZIP CODE, COUNTRY	TYPE ESTABLISHMENT INSPECTED
Blakely, GA 39823-1881	Peanut Roaster/Peanut Butter and Paste Manufacturer

boxes utilizing a hopper in the "kitchen area", this location is where the raw peanuts enter the roaster, again no segregation. Raw peanuts are filled into boxes utilizing a hopper located in the Production/Packaging room. This hopper is positioned above the packaging line for the small party packs of roasted peanuts. There is no segregation of raw and finished product in this area.

OBSERVATION 8

Devices and fixtures are not designed and constructed to protect against recontamination of clean, sanitized hands.

Specifically, the sink located in the peanut butter room is used interchangeably as a point for cleaning hands and utensils and for washing out mops.

OBSERVATION 9

Failure to conduct cleaning and sanitizing operations for utensils and equipment in a manner that protects against contamination of food.

Specifically, on 1/12/09 a build-up of product residue was observed on grinders, hoppers, and support beams on the peanut paste tanker line. Also, pieces of the yellow and black caution sign on th (b)(4) mill were flaking off into the catch pan for product under the mill.

On 1/9/09, the dry ingredient staging area above the peanut butter room was dirty with a heavy build-up of different powdery ingredients on all exposed surfaces. This is an open area of the ceiling located directly above the dry ingredient hopper and ribbon mixer.

On 1/9/09, a mesh-type conveyor was observed to be stored in the firm's equipment/utensil wash room, which was used as a catch-all storage area for buckets, stainless steel pipes, removable pumps, removable Y-spouts, and floor mats. The insides and end rollers of this conveyor were covered with a slimy, black-brown residue. Additionally, the bottom sections of the wash room walls had areas of mold.

AMENDED

	EMPLOYEE(S) SIGNATURE	DATE ISSUED
SEE REVERSE OF THIS PAGE	Janet B Gray, Investigator Darcy E. Brillhart, Microbiologist Sandra T. Saul, Investigator Robert P. Neligan, Investigator Lesley K. Satterwhite, Microbiologist Theresa L. Stewart, Investigator	02/05/2009

FORM FDA 483 (04/03) PREVIOUS EDITION OBSOLETE INSPECTIONAL OBSERVATIONS PAGE 7 OF 8 PAGES

DEPARTMENT OF HEALTH AND HUMAN SERVICES
FOOD AND DRUG ADMINISTRATION

DISTRICT ADDRESS AND PHONE NUMBER	DATE(S) OF INSPECTION
60 Eighth Street NE Atlanta, GA 30309 (404) 253-1161 Fax:(404) 253-1202 Industry Information: www.fda.gov/oc/industry	01/09/2009 - 02/05/2009* FEI NUMBER 1036857

NAME AND TITLE OF INDIVIDUAL TO WHOM REPORT ISSUED
TO: Sammy L. Lightsey, Plant Operations Manager

FIRM NAME	STREET ADDRESS
Peanut Corporation Of America	14075 Magnolia St.
CITY, STATE, ZIP CODE, COUNTRY	TYPE ESTABLISHMENT INSPECTED
Blakely, GA 39823-1881	Peanut Roaster/Peanut Butter and Paste Manufacturer

OBSERVATION 10

Effective measures are not being taken to protect against the contamination of food on the premises by pests.

Specifically, on 1/9/09 a live roach and several dead roaches were observed in the firm's wash room. This wash room is adjacent to the production/packaging area.

Also, the bumper pads used for sealing the trailers against the bay doors were inadequate in that openings of 6 inches or more were observed along the sides and tops of the trailers. These trailers, containing raw or roasted product in totes, can be left backed up to the bay doors for 5-7 days allowing these openings to exist.

*** DATES OF INSPECTION:**
01/09/2009(Fri), 01/12/2009(Mon), 01/13/2009(Tue), 01/14/2009(Wed), 01/15/2009(Thu), 01/16/2009(Fri), 01/19/2009(Mon), 01/20/2009(Tue), 01/21/2009(Wed), 01/22/2009(Thu), 01/23/2009(Fri), 01/26/2009(Mon), 01/27/2009(Tue), 02/05/2009(Thu)

AMENDED

	EMPLOYEE(S) SIGNATURE	DATE ISSUED
SEE REVERSE OF THIS PAGE	Janet B Gray, Investigator Darcy E. Brillhart, Microbiologist Sandra I. Gaul, Investigator Robert P. Neligan, Investigator Lesley K. Satterwhite, Microbiologist Theresa L. Stewart, Investigator	02/05/2009

FORM FDA 483 (04/03) PREVIOUS EDITION OBSOLETE INSPECTIONAL OBSERVATIONS PAGE 5 OF 5 PAGES

In: The Salmonella Outbreak in Peanut Products: The FDA … ISBN: 978-1-60741-950-1
Editor: Benjamin K. Glynn

Chapter 10

THE FDA'S AUTHORITY TO RECALL PRODUCTS

Vanessa K. Burrows

SUMMARY

The Food and Drug Administration (FDA) has fielded increasing numbers of questions regarding recalls of unsafe imports, including jalapeño peppers, pet food, the blood thinner heparin, and toothpaste. Additionally, several domestic food products, from peanut butter contaminated with *Salmonella* to spinach linked to *E. coli 015 7:H7* to canned meat products such as chili sauce spoiled by *Clostridium botulinum* (botulism), have been voluntarily recalled by businesses in the last year. Recalls may decrease consumer confidence in the recalling company, food imports, or food safety agencies such as the FDA; products later subject to a recall may have sickened or killed people or pets. While the FDA only has the authority to order recalls of infant formula, medical devices, and human tissue products, the agency may request that a company recall other products, such as food, drugs, and cosmetics. This report provides an overview of the FDA's statutory authority with regard to the three types of products that it can recall, as well as FDA regulations for designating the particular class of recall, publicizing and monitoring the effectiveness of recalls, and carrying out recalls. Additionally, this report reviews the recall provisions in legislation proposed in the 110th Congress, which would give the FDA authority to require recalls of additional products.

The 110th Congress has shown significant interest in the issue of food safety. Congress passed H.R. 3580, P.L. 110-85, the FDA Amendments Act of 2007 (FDAAA), which contains provisions addressing communications and information postings during a food recall similar to those the Senate previously approved, by a vote of 94-0, in Senator Durbin's amendment to the FDA Revitalization Act (S. 1082/H.R. 2900). Several bills would grant the FDA the ability to order recalls of food and other products. The Food and Drug Import Safety Act of 2007, H.R. 3610, would grant the Secretary of Health and Human Services (HHS) the authority to require food recalls. Representative Dingell's draft of the Food and Drug Administration Globalization Act of 2008 — posted for comment on the House Energy and Commerce Committee web site — would also grant the Secretary the authority to require food recalls and, in addition, would grant the Secretary the same authority for recalling drugs as the Secretary has for recalling devices. The Family Smoking Prevention and Tobacco Control Act, S. 625/H.R. 1108, would provide the Secretary with the authority to require recalls of tobacco products. Other bills that would provide the FDA with recall authority include the FDA Food Safety Modernization Act, S. 3385; the Human and Pet Food Safety Act of 2007, S. 1274/H.R. 2108; the Safe Food Act of 2007, S. 654/H.R. 1148; the Protect Consumers Act of 2007, H.R. 2099; the Safe And Fair Enforcement and Recall for (SAFER) Meat, Poultry, and Food Act of 2007, H.R. 3484; the Food and Product Responsibility Act of 2007, S. 2081; the Consumer Food Safety Act of 2007, H.R. 3624; and the Food Import Safety Act of 2007, H.R. 3937.

Background

The Food and Drug Administration (FDA) has fielded increasing numbers of questions regarding recalls of unsafe imports, including jalapeño peppers, pet food, the blood thinner heparin, and toothpaste. Additionally, several domestic food products, from peanut butter contaminated with *Salmonella* to spinach linked to *E. coli 015 7:H7* to canned meat products such as chili sauce spoiled by *Clostridium botulinum* (botulism), have been recalled in the last year. A recall is "a firm's removal or correction of a marketed product that the [FDA] considers to be in violation of the laws it administers and against which the agency would initiate legal action, e.g., seizure."[1]

Recalls may decrease consumer confidence in the recalling company, food imports, or food safety agencies such as the FDA; products later subject to a recall may have sickened or killed people or pets.[2] Recalls of tainted or defective products can be costly to the recalling company in terms of the costs of the recall, injury to reputation, and exposure to liability via class action lawsuits and punitive damages.[3] For example, pet owners filed suit against Menu Foods seeking "compensation for veterinary care, medical monitoring and other expenses, damages for negligence and breach of express and implied warranty and attorney fees and costs," which reportedly may settle for $24 million.[4] The company began testing its pet food on animals at the end of February 2007, "one week after it began hearing from owners who said the food had made their pets ill."[5] However, the company did not contact the FDA or begin a recall of more than 60 million containers of pet food until March 2007.[6]

While the FDA only has the authority to order recalls of infant formula, medical devices, and human tissue products, the agency may request that a company voluntarily recall other products, such as food, drugs, and cosmetics. Companies typically recall tainted products voluntarily but this may not always be the case.[7] For this reason and others discussed below, supporters of stronger food safety laws have argued that the FDA should be given statutory authority to mandate recalls of food and other products.

This report provides an overview of the FDA's statutory authority with regard to the three types of products for which the agency can require recalls, as well as FDA regulations for designating the particular class of recall, publicizing and monitoring the effectiveness of recalls, and carrying out recalls. Additionally, this report reviews the recall provisions in legislation proposed in the 110th Congress, which would give the FDA authority to require recalls of additional products.

Mandatory Recall Authority: Supporting and Opposing Views

Representative Rosa DeLauro and others have reportedly asserted that the current food safety system, which "relies on voluntary recalls[,] implicitly protects industry before it protects public health."[8] As a result, some argue that the discovery of the source of contaminated products may not immediately be identified.[9] The FDA has also been accused of failing to aggressively pursue investigations of products that were later recalled.[10] For example, lawsuits have been brought against ConAgra Foods, Inc. by individuals who allegedly became sick, sometimes more than once, because they ate peanut butter tainted with *Salmonella*. According to the plaintiffs, ConAgra did not recall contaminated peanut butter from one plant until February 2007, though the FDA "suspected that peanut butter manufactured by ConAgra Foods under different brand names might have been contaminated with salmonella" as early as 2005.[11]

Consumer rights groups seek new statutory authority that would allow the FDA to mandate recalls of food and other products.[12] However, the FDA's Center for Food Safety and Applied Nutrition has argued that "cooperation between FDA and its regulated industries has proven over the years to be the quickest and most reliable method to remove potentially dangerous products from the market."[13] According to the agency, both the FDA and industry share an interest in removing unsafe and/or defective products from the marketplace.[14] An industry representative involved in the pet food recall has also argued against additional regulation, saying that industry "could have been a more valuable partner" in the recall process if it received access to the same information as the FDA.[15] According to the head of the Pet Food Institute, which represents U.S. pet food manufacturers, the communication of such information would have allowed the organization to "cross-reference . . . lot numbers, shipping information, and other data."[16]

Some have argued that in situations where the manufacturer of a product cannot be determined — such as the case of tainted toothpaste found in discount stores, prisons, hospitals, and luxury hotels — granting the FDA the ability to recall such products would expedite the process of removing adulterated articles from store shelves.[17] Such authority would enable the agency to take actions beyond issuing a warning about a particular product.[18] A 2004 Government Accountability Office (GAO) report found that:

> FDA do[es] not know how promptly and completely the recalling companies and their distributors and other customers are carrying out recalls, and neither [the FDA nor the U.S. Department of Agriculture (USDA)] is using its data systems to effectively track and manage its recall programs. For these and other reasons, most recalled food is not recovered and therefore may be consumed.[19]

According to GAO, the FDA may not be using the regulations on voluntary recalls that the agency currently has in place to their maximum effectiveness.[20] The staff of the House Energy and Commerce Committee's Subcommittee on Oversight and Investigations has also remarked that the "FDA's current regulatory approach, which relies upon voluntary guidelines for most domestic and imported foods, appears inadequate in responding to the changing food industry."[21]

In addition, advocates for a single food safety agency argue that a single contact point could save time and lives in the event of a food recall.[22] As demonstrated by the chili products recall due to the potential for botulism, more than one agency may have jurisdiction over adulterated or contaminated food.[23] In that situation, the FDA website listed all the recalled product numbers but only included photos of the labels for chili products that did not contain meat and pet food products involved in the same recall. (The FDA has jurisdiction over pet food.) Consumers were directed to the USDA Meat and Poultry Hotline website for products containing meat, over which the USDA has jurisdiction.[24] The linked USDA webpage provides general information, but does not provide information about the meat products recalled due to being potentially contaminated with botulism.[25] Some have argued that the lack of complete information regarding the recall, as well as links to webpages not specifically associated with the chili product recall, could result in consumers overlooking relevant information and potentially consuming tainted products. The Food Marketing Institute — a nonprofit association of retailers and wholesalers that account for the majority of U.S. grocery store sales — and others have contended that the creation of a single food safety agency would help in a food crisis, because the "public is faced with a lengthy delay while overlapping bureaucracies creak into some attempt at a coordinated response. While the search for who knew what and when goes on, the crisis worsens and public confidence erodes."[26]

Those opposed to the idea of combining FDA and USDA into a single food safety agency assert that such a measure would distract the agencies involved from their mission while the reorganization process occurs.[27] They argue that "food security would be compromised" and that overlap between agencies "is not as significant [an issue] as many assume."[28] Furthermore, critics of a single food safety agency point out that coordination between federal, state, and local government agencies would still be required to address threats to the food supply.[29]

Current Statutory Authority for Mandatory Recalls

The FDA possesses mandatory recall authority only with regard to three products: infant formula,[30] medical devices,[31] and biologic products.[32] This section provides an overview of the statutory authorities that exist for recalling these three products. The FDA is one of several agencies that comprise HHS. Therefore, the Federal Food, Drug, and Cosmetic Act (FFDCA) provisions refer to the Secretary of HHS, who, in turn, delegates authority to the FDA.

Infant Formula

The HHS Secretary has prescribed regulations for recalls of infant formula "begun by a manufacturer,"[33] which address the mandatory scope and extent of infant formula recalls "necessary and appropriate for the degree of risks to human health presented by the formula subject to the recall."[34] The regulations for infant formula recalls are available at 21 C.F.R. Part 107, Subpart E, Infant Formula Recalls, and state, in part, the following:

> When the Food and Drug Administration determines that an adulterated or misbranded infant formula presents a risk to human health, a manufacturer shall immediately take all actions necessary to recall that formula, extending to and including the retail level, consistent with the requirements of [21 C.F.R. Part 107, Subpart E].[35]

The FFDCA states that the regulations must require manufacturers that begin an infant formula recall "because of a risk to human health to request each retail establishment at which such formula is sold or available for sale to post at the point of purchase . . . a notice of such recall at such establishment for such time that the Secretary determines necessary to inform the public of such recall."[36] The FFDCA also requires manufacturers of infant formula to create and keep "records respecting the distribution of infant formula through any establishment owned or operated by such manufacturer as may be necessary to effect and monitor recalls."[37] The manufacturer must retain such records for "at least one year after the expiration of the shelf life of the infant formula,"[38] and the Secretary may promulgate regulations regarding recordkeeping if the Secretary determines that the required records "are not being made or maintained."[39]

Medical Devices

The FFDCA's medical device recall authority provisions place requirements on device manufacturers, importers, distributors, retailers, and other "appropriate persons." If the HHS Secretary "finds that there is a reasonable probability that a device intended for human use would cause serious, adverse health consequences or death," then the Secretary must issue an order requiring "the appropriate person" to (1) immediately stop distributing the device, (2) immediately notify health professionals and device user facilities of the Secretary's order, and (3) instruct health professionals and device user facilities to stop use of the device.[40] Thus, the first step of the statute does not require a mandatory recall of a device for which the Secretary makes the above determination.

However, the order may be amended to mandate a recall of such device. The Secretary's order must "provide the person subject to the order with an opportunity for an informal hearing, to be held not later than 10 days after the date of the issuance of the order, on the actions required by the order and on whether the order should be amended to require a recall."[41] If the Secretary determines, after the informal hearing, that the order should be amended as such, the Secretary must amend the order to require the recall, set a timetable for the recall, and require periodic reports describing the recall's progress.[42] The Secretary's amended order must not include a recall of the device from individuals and must not include a recall from device user facilities "if the Secretary determines that the risk of recalling such device from the facilities presents a greater health risk than the health risk of not recalling the device from use."[43]

Additionally, the Secretary's amended order must provide "notice to individuals subject to the risks associated with the use of such device."[44] To notify individuals regarding the device, the statute provides that "the Secretary may use the assistance of health professionals who prescribed or used such a device."[45] However, if "a significant number" of individuals cannot be identified, the Secretary must notify them via FFDCA § 705(b). That provision gives the Secretary the broad authority to "cause to be disseminated information . . . in situations involving, in the opinion of the Secretary, imminent danger to health, or gross deception of the consumer."[46] Recalling a device is only one of the methods that the Secretary may use to address the risk it presents to the public health. The Secretary may also notify health professionals who prescribe or use the device; order the manufacturer, importer, or any distributor to submit a plan for repairing or replacing the device, or refunding all or part of the purchase cost of the device; and may require the manufacturer, importer, distributor, or retailer to reimburse, for expenses incurred in carrying out the Secretary's order, "any other person who is a manufacturer, importer, distributor, or retailer."[47]

Biological Products

For biological products such as blood, blood components, and human tissue, the Secretary must issue an order immediately requiring a recall of "a batch, lot, or other quantity of a product licensed under [42 U.S.C. § 262, Regulation of Biological Products]" once a determination is made that that quantity "presents an imminent or substantial hazard to the public health."[48] The Secretary's order must be issued in accordance with 5 U.S.C. § 554, which addresses formal adjudications after an opportunity for an agency hearing. Violators of these provisions may face inflation-adjustable civil penalties of up to $100,000 per day of violation.[49]

Current FDA Regulations Regarding Voluntary Recalls

Part 7, Subpart C, of Title 21, Code of Federal Regulations gives "guidance for manufacturers and distributors to follow with respect to their voluntary removal or correction" of a FDA-regulated product on the market that violates the FFDCA or other law that the FDA administers.[50] Chapter Seven of the FDA's Regulatory Procedures Manual also serves as a reference for FDA employees and industry as to recall procedures; the manual is not law and does not bind the FDA or industry.[51] As a result, only FDA regulatory authorities and not the manual are discussed in this report.

The FDA views voluntary, industry-initiated recalls as an alternative to FDA legal actions to remove or correct products that violate laws.[52] For example, the FDA has the power to seize adulterated and misbranded products under the FFDCA.[53] However, the agency states that a company recall "is generally more appropriate and affords better protection for consumers than seizure, when many lots of the product have been widely distributed."[54] The FDA may turn to seizure as a remedy if "the agency has reason to believe that a recall would not be effective, determines that a recall is ineffective, or discovers that a violation is continuing."[55]

Industry-Initiated Recalls

The FDA recommends that companies undertake certain practices that may prepare them for a recall or assist them during a recall. These include (1) creating a contingency plan, (2) using codes on FDA-regulated products that will make it possible to identify and recall the defective products, and (3) keeping records — even beyond the shelf or expected use life of a product — that can be used to find the tainted products.[56] If a company initiates a recall, the FDA regulations suggest that the firm immediately notify the closest FDA district office. If the product being recalled would be subject to a court action, such as seizure for being misbranded or adulterated, then the FDA deems the company's action to be a recall and will ask the business to provide the agency with information on the amount and identity of the product, as well as communications about the recall and other data.[57]

FDA regulations also provide for instances in which a company decides to recall a product after being informed by the agency that "the product in question violates the law, but the agency has not specifically requested a recall."[58] In this case, the company's decision to recall the product is treated as an industry-initiated recall. Furthermore, agency regulations provide procedures if a company begins to remove or correct a product in a way that the company believes would constitute a market withdrawal. A market withdrawal is "a firm's removal or correction of a distributed product which involves a minor violation that would not be subject to legal action by the [FDA] or which involves no violation, e.g., normal stock rotation practices."[59] If the business is conducting a market withdrawal, but the reason for the need to remove the product is not clear, the FDA is willing to help the company ascertain the cause of the problem. For example, consumers may have experienced adverse reactions to the product, but the source of the problem may not be "obvious or clearly understood."[60]

FDA-Requested Recalls

The FDA can request a business to voluntarily recall a FDA-regulated product; however, such requests are "reserved for urgent situations."[61] The FDA would make such a request to the company with "primary responsibility for the manufacture and marketing" of the defective product.[62] The FDA Commissioner can request a company to conduct a recall after these three determinations have been made:

1. That a product that has been distributed presents a risk of illness or injury or gross consumer deception.
2. That the firm has not initiated a recall of the product.
3. That an agency action is necessary to protect public health and welfare.[63]

If the company refuses to recall its products after the FDA makes its request, the agency may then turn to seizures or other court actions to protect the public health.[64] According to its regulations, if the FDA requests a recall, the agency should take into account the factors listed in its recall strategy, such as "the degree to which the product remains unused in the marketplace" and the "ease in identifying the product."[65]

Classification of Recalls

The FDA categorizes recalls in three classes. Class I recalls involve "situation[s] in which there is a reasonable probability that the use of, or exposure to, a violative product will cause serious adverse health consequences or death."[66] According to the FDA, over 100 Class I recalls of food products occurred in FY2006 and the average number of Class I food recalls for the last five fiscal years is 188.[67] Class II recalls involve "situation[s] in which use of, or exposure to, a violative product may cause temporary or medically reversible adverse health consequences or where the probability of serious adverse health consequences is remote," while Class III recalls involve "situation[s] in which use of, or exposure to, a violative product is not likely to cause adverse health consequences."[68] The FDA posts information regarding all three classes of recalls on its website in the agency's weekly FDA Enforcement Report.[69] Additionally, the FDA's webpage devoted to "Recalls, Market Withdrawals, and Safety Alerts" contains press releases and information for mostly Class I recalls.[70]

In order to determine what classification to assign a recall, an ad hoc committee of FDA scientists, perhaps at the closest FDA district office, will first examine the factors below.

1. Whether any disease or injuries have already occurred from the use of the product.
2. Whether any existing conditions could contribute to a clinical situation that could expose humans or animals to a health hazard. Any conclusion shall be supported as completely as possible by scientific documentation and/or statements that the conclusion is the opinion of the individual(s) making the health hazard determination.
3. Assessment of hazard to various segments of the population, e.g., children, surgical patients, pets, livestock, etc., who are expected to be exposed to the product being considered, with particular attention paid to the hazard to those individuals who may be at greatest risk.
4. Assessment of the degree of seriousness of the health hazard to which the populations at risk would be exposed.
5. Assessment of the likelihood of occurrence of the hazard.
6. Assessment of the consequences (immediate or long-range) of occurrence of the hazard.[71]

The committee is not limited to evaluating the health hazard posed by a product based on these factors alone however.[72] The FDA is to then use the committee's health hazard evaluation as the basis for assigning a classification.[73]

Communication Regarding a Recall

The company that recalls a product "is responsible for promptly notifying each of its affected direct accounts about the recall."[74] The FDA regulations set out what information should be specified in the notification, such as the identity of the product, the need to stop distributing the product, that the notified person should in turn notify its customers, and what other steps to take with the recalled product. The agency also provides instructions about the contents — or lack thereof, in the case of including promotional materials that could distract from the recall information — and appearance of the communication that will inform a customer of the recall. Those who purchased, received, or used the product being recalled who are notified via a recall communication should also promptly notify their customers or the individuals who may have received or used the product.[75] As mentioned above, the FDA will place information regarding recalls in its weekly FDA Enforcement Report, with two exceptions: (1) product removals or corrections that the FDA finds are market withdrawals or stock recoveries[76] and (2) "intentionally delay[ed] public notification of recalls of certain drugs and devices where the agency determines that public notification may cause unnecessary and harmful anxiety in patients and that initial consultation between patients and their physicians is essential."[77]

Monitoring and Termination of a Recall

The FDA regulations request that companies recalling products to send progress reports on the recall to the appropriate FDA district or field office. The FDA is to inform the firm, based on the urgency of the recall, of how often it should submit recall status reports.[78] The recalling company should continue to send recall progress reports until the FDA terminates the recall, and such reports should include information on the numbers of individuals who were notified, who responded, or who failed to respond to the company's recall communication. The reports should also state the number of products returned and accounted for, how many verification checks were conducted to determine if the recall was effective and the results of such checks, and the firm's estimate of the time until the recall is completed.[79] The FDA field office "is responsible for determining whether the recall was effective and that disposition of the product was completed properly."[80]

Once the FDA "determines that all reasonable efforts have been made to remove or correct the product in accordance with the recall strategy, and when it is reasonable to assume that the product subject to the recall has been removed" and either disposed of or corrected, the agency is to issue a written notice that the recall is terminated.[81] The FDA's determination may depend on the degree of public health hazard associated with product being recalled.[82] For Class I recalls, the FDA district office is to prepare a recommendation for the appropriate FDA center, such as the Center for Food Safety and Applied Nutrition, that the Class I recall be terminated. However, Class II and III recalls do not need approval from an FDA Center.[83] Alternately, the recalling company can request, in writing, that the FDA terminate the recall. This request should include a statement in writing that the recall is effective, in line with the type of determination that the FDA would make when terminating a recall.[84] The FDA's Regulatory Procedures Manual states that the time from when a company considers its recall complete to the time when the agency terminates the recall should generally not exceed three months.[85]

The FDA's Pilot Program

From mid-February 2007 until August 12, 2007, the FDA ran a six-month pilot program "to educate and assist consumers in identifying recalled food products that may pose a significant health risk."[86] The program concentrated on posting photos of Class I food product recalls, in the hope that pictures of the main label or display panel would help consumers recognize and avoid using recalled products. Press releases with these photos also contained other identifying information for the food product, such as a lot number or flavor of a product, if only one flavor was affected.[87] The FDA accepted comments from consumers and industry on the program, and the agency's website stated that the program would be "continuing for a short time after the end date while it is being evaluated."[88]

Food and Drug Administration Amendments Act of 2007 (FDAAA)

Public Law 110-85 contains provisions addressing communications and information postings during a food recall.[89] To enhance communication during a recall, the law requires the Secretary to post information regarding recalled human or pet food products on the FDA website; work with industry, professional organizations, and others to gather information relevant to the recall; and communicate with the public.[90] The law mandates that the HHS Secretary, by September 27, 2008, "establish an early warning and surveillance system to identify adulteration of the pet food supply and outbreaks of illness associated with pet food."[91] The law also requires the Secretary to work with notification networks during a pet food recall "to inform veterinarians and relevant stakeholders."[92]

Legislative Proposals to Grant the FDA Recall Authority

The 110th Congress has shown significant interest in the issue of food safety. Several bills would grant the FDA the ability to order recalls of food products, drugs, and tobacco products. The following summaries of proposed legislation address the mandatory recall provisions in such legislation. S. 2418, the Ending Agricultural Threats: Safeguarding America's Food for Everyone (EAT SAFE) Act of 2007 also contains provisions regarding product recalls; however, it does not provide the FDA with mandatory recall authority.

Human and Pet Food Safety Act of 2007

S. 1274 and H.R. 2108 propose to amend the FFDCA to allow the HHS Secretary to handle recalls in a voluntary manner at first. The bills would give the Secretary statutory authority for both voluntary and mandatory recalls. If the Secretary determines that food in interstate commerce violates the FFDCA and "that there is a reasonable probability that the food, if consumed, would present a threat to public health," the bills then require the

Secretary to "give the appropriate persons (including the manufacturers, importers, distributors, or retailers of the food) an opportunity to" cease distributing the food; notify individuals such as distributors, processors, handlers, consumers, and state and local public health officials; and recall the food.[93] The bills also provide civil penalties of up to $10,000 per violation per day.[94]

If a person, such as a manufacturer, refuses to or fails to adequately carry out the above described actions "within the time period and in the manner prescribed by the Secretary," the bills would grant the Secretary the authority to "control and possess the food, including ordering the shipment of the food from a food establishment . . . to the Secretary" at either the establishment's expense or, in an emergency, at the Secretary's expense.[95] The Secretary would be required to issue an order mandating importers, retailers, or others to stop distributing the food and notify those involved with the food product's handling, transportation, sale, and other activities. Furthermore, the Secretary must notify "consumers to whom the food was, or may have been distributed," as well as state and local public health officials.[96] Persons such as distributors, processors, handlers, and sellers notified by either the Secretary or an "appropriate person," as described above, must also stop distributing the food product and make available records regarding others who processed, distributed, and sold the food.[97] After an informal hearing, the Secretary would also be able to require a recall, set a timetable for the recall, mandate progress reports on the recall, and give notice of the recall to consumers.[98]

The bills also contain provisions similar to those incorporated in FDAAA. To enhance communication during a recall, the bills would require the Secretary to post information regarding recalled human or pet food products on the FDA website; work with industry, professional organizations, and others to gather information relevant to the recall; and communicate with the public.[99] Finally, the HHS Secretary would have to work with notification networks during a pet food recall "to inform veterinarians and relevant stakeholders."[100]

Food and Drug Administration Revitalization Act

Senator Durbin's amendment to S. 1082, which passed 94-0, contains the same communication and notification requirements during recalls as the Human and Pet Food Safety Act of 2007 (see above), which were similar to those incorporated in FDAAA. The amendment would expand the FDA's authority in other areas as well.

Safe Food Act of 2007

S. 654 and H.R. 1148 would create an independent single food agency, headed by an Administrator of Food Safety. The bills' voluntary and mandatory recall provisions, in Section 403, are basically the same as those in the Human and Pet Food Safety Act of 2007, except that the Administrator replaces the Secretary of HHS; the term "food establishment" is defined in these bills;[101] and S. 654 and H.R. 1148 prohibit violations of food safety laws in general — from the Egg Products Inspection Act to the Sanitary Food Transportation Act of 1990, as amended — rather than solely the FFDCA.

The bills would institute additional recall provisions as well. Section 204 of the bills would give the Administrator the power to order recalls from food establishments if the Administrator determines that an establishment fails to meet a performance standard for contaminants in food and does not take corrective actions determined by the Administrator. These standards would be promulgated by the Administrator. The frequency with which a food establishment conducts recalls of its products would be taken into account in the bills' provisions classifying food establishments and how often the new agency would inspect such establishments.[102] The bills also specify that any protections that the Administrator develops "to prevent the unauthorized disclosure of any trade secret or confidential information obtained by the Administrator" would not "limit the public disclosure of distribution records or other records related to a food subject to a voluntary or mandatory recall."[103] Section 207 of the bills states that the new agency's Administrator must support state and local recall authorities. Like the current FFDCA, the bills create a section of prohibited acts, one of which would be failing to comply with a recall or other order.[104] Additionally, the bills provide civil and criminal penalties.[105]

FDA Food Safety Modernization Act

Under S. 3385, the Secretary must first provide the responsible party with an opportunity to voluntarily cease distribution and recall the article of food if the Secretary makes a determination based on information gathered through the FFDCA reportable food registry or through any other means. The Secretary may determine that there is a reasonable probability that an article of food is adulterated or misbranded, and the use of or exposure to such article will cause serious adverse health consequences or death to humans or animals. If a person refuses to comply or does not voluntarily comply with a request by the Secretary to cease distribution or sale of, or to recall, an article of food, the Secretary would be authorized to issue an order to cease distribution and to immediately notify others to stop distribution of the article of food. After an opportunity for an informal hearing, the Secretary could amend the order to cease distribution to include a mandatory recall of the food involved, set a timetable for the recall, require reports on its progress from the responsible party, and provide notice to consumers to whom the food may have been distributed.

The Secretary would be required to work with state and local public health officials, as appropriate, to carry out the recall provisions of the bill. In conducting a recall, the Secretary would be required to issue a press release, and other notices as appropriate, to provide consumers and retailers with information about the affected articles of food, and the risks posed. The Secretary's authority to issue or vacate recall orders would not be able to be delegated to anyone other than the FDA Commissioner, and the bill's recall provisions would not affect the authority of the Secretary to request or participate in a voluntary recall. Failure to comply with an order by the Secretary would be a prohibited act under the FFDCA, and the person who does not comply with such an order would be subject to a civil monetary penalty.

Protect Consumers Act of 2007

H.R. 2099 would enable the HHS Secretary to institute a mandatory recall of an FDA-regulated product. Under the bill, if the Secretary makes a determination that a mandatory recall is necessary, the Secretary must issue an order requiring distribution, manufacture, and sales of the product to cease; giving "notice to individuals subject to the risks associated with the use of such product"; and recalling the product immediately.[106] The bill would provide for an opportunity for an informal hearing after the order is issued. Depending on whether the Secretary determines that there are adequate grounds to support the order, the order could be vacated or could remain in effect until a future decision by the Secretary. Noncompliance with an order would be treated as a violation of the FFDCA. Section 3 of the bill would also provide for a study on procedures for instituting voluntary and mandatory recalls and making them more effective. The Secretary would also be required to promulgate regulations as a result of the study on new recall procedures.

Food and Drug Import Safety Act of 2007

Section 10 of H.R. 3610 would grant the FDA mandatory authority to order manufacturers, importers, distributors, retailers, and others to stop distributing food products if "the Secretary finds that a food may cause serious, adverse health consequences or death." After an opportunity for an informal hearing, the HHS Secretary could amend the order to cease distribution to include a mandatory recall of the food involved, except from individuals. The Secretary would also set a timetable for the recall and require reports on its progress. This proposal has been endorsed by the consumer group Food & Water Watch, which believes that "giving FDA such authority will speed up the removal of adulterated food from commerce."[107]

Food and Product Responsibility Act of 2007

S. 2081 would grant the FDA authority, after the Secretary has provided an opportunity for an informal hearing, to require a recall of an article of food if "the Secretary determines that there is a reasonable probability that human consumption of the article . . . presents a threat to public health." After an opportunity for an informal hearing, the HHS Secretary may also set a timetable for the recall, require reports on its progress, and "provide notice of the recall to consumers to which the article was, or may have been, distributed." The bill would also require manufacturers of food, drugs, devices, cosmetics, biologics, meat and poultry and their products, consumer products, eggs and egg products, and certain replacement equipment to obtain a recall responsibility certificate from U.S. Customs and Border Protection that indicates

> a manufacturer possess[es] sufficient means (through insurance or otherwise) for the 5-year period beginning on the date the manufacturer begins to distribute in commerce [such a] product, to cover — (A) the entire cost of a recall of that product . . . ; and (B) compensatory

damages and costs (including reasonable attorneys fees) of any product liability or other lawsuit filed for claims arising out of, relating to, or resulting from any defect in that product.

SAFER Meat, Poultry, and Food Act of 2007

H.R. 3484 would grant the FDA authority to mandate a recall of an article of food if the Secretary finds that it is "adulterated or misbranded in a manner that, if consumed, may result in illness or injury." The Secretary must first provide an opportunity for a person to take voluntary actions such as recalling the article of food or stopping distribution of the article. Then, if the person "does not carry out the actions . . . within the time period and in the manner prescribed by the Secretary," the Secretary must require the immediate ceasing of distribution of the article of food, including the immediate notification of others to stop distribution of the article of food. The Secretary may also "take control or possession of the article," which would be in addition to the Secretary's existing seizure authority under FFDCA § 304, and notify consumers and state and local health officials. The Secretary must provide an opportunity for a hearing on an order issued by the Secretary, and, after such hearing, may amend the order to require a recall of an article of food or other action, set a timetable for the recall, require reports on the recall's progress, and "provide notice of the recall to consumers to which the article was, or may have been, distributed," if the Secretary determines that the article "is adulterated or misbranded in a manner that, if consumed, may result in illness or injury."

The bill would also make it a prohibited act under the FFDCA to fail to comply with certain orders or an amended order issued by the Secretary, such as those that would require a person to cease distribution of an article of food or would require a recall of the article of food. H.R. 3484 would also increase civil penalties for those who commit prohibited acts "with respect to an article of food" and make "[e]ach prohibited act and each day during which the act continues . . . a separate offense."

Consumer Food Safety Act of 2007

H.R. 3624 contains provisions similar to H.R. 3484. H.R. 3624 would grant the FDA authority to mandate a recall of an article of food if the Secretary finds that it is "adulterated or misbranded" and "there is a reasonable probability that such article, if consumed, would present a threat to public health." The Secretary must first provide an opportunity for a person to take voluntary actions such as recalling the article of food or stopping distribution of the article. Then, if the person "refuses to or does not voluntarily cease distribution, make notification, recall such article, or provide notice to consumers, as applicable, within the time and in the manner prescribed by the Secretary," the Secretary must require the immediate ceasing of distribution of the article of food, or the immediate notification of others, such as those who process and transport the article of food, or both actions. The Secretary also "shall, as the Secretary deems necessary, provide notice to consumers to whom such article was, or may have been distributed." The Secretary must provide an opportunity for a hearing on an order issued by the Secretary, and after such hearing, may amend the order to require a recall of an article of food or other action, set a timetable for the recall, require reports on the recall's progress, and "provide notice of the recall to consumers to which the article was, or may have been, distributed," if the Secretary determines that "there is a reasonable probability that the article . . . if consumed, presents a threat to public health."

The bill would make the failure to comply with certain orders or an amended order issued by the Secretary, such as those that would require a person to cease distribution of an article of food or would require a recall of the article of food, a prohibited act under the FFDCA. H.R. 3624 would add civil penalties for those who commit a violation of the FFDCA or the Consumer Food Safety Act of 2007 with respect to food. H.R. 3624 would also enable any person to sue for a violation of a recall order or "other action of the Secretary to ensure the safety of food products."

Food Import Safety Act of 2007

Under H.R. 3937, the Secretary must first provide an opportunity for a person to take voluntary actions such as recalling the article of food or stopping distribution of the article, if the Secretary has determined that the food violates the FFDCA and "that there is a reasonable probability that the food, if consumed, would present a threat to public health." Then, if the person "refuses to or does not adequately carry out the action described . . . within the time period and in the manner prescribed by the Secretary," H.R. 3937 would grant the FDA authority to "control and possess the food, including ordering the shipment of the food from a food establishment," or to require a person to immediately cease distribution of the food and notify others with regard to the immediate ceasing of distribution of the food. The Secretary also "shall, as the Secretary deems necessary, provide notice . . . to consumers to whom the food was, or may have been, distributed" and to state and local public health officials. The Secretary must provide an opportunity for an informal hearing on an order issued by the Secretary, and after such hearing, may amend the order to require a recall of an article of food or other action, set a timetable for the recall, require reports on the recall's progress, and "provide notice of the recall to consumers to which the article was, or may have been, distributed," if the Secretary determines that "there is a reasonable probability that the food . . . if consumed, would present a threat to public health."

The bill would also add civil penalties for those who violate its notification and recall standards. Each violative act and each day a violation continues would be considered a separate offense, and the bill provides for a good faith exception to the civil penalties.

Draft of the Food and Drug Administration Globalization Act of 2008

On the website of the House Energy and Commerce Committee, Representative Dingell has posted a discussion draft of a bill that would be entitled the Food and Drug Administration Globalization Act of 2008.[108] The bill would grant the Secretary the authority to require food recalls and would grant the Secretary the same authority for recalling drugs as the Secretary has for recalling devices.

Family Smoking Prevention and Tobacco Control Act

S. 625 and H.R. 1108 would provide the HHS Secretary with the authority to require recalls of tobacco products in a manner substantially similar to the Secretary's authority to recall medical devices. "If the Secretary finds that there is a reasonable probability that a tobacco product contains a manufacturing or other defect not ordinarily contained in tobacco products on the market that would cause serious, adverse health consequences or death," then the Secretary must issue an order requiring distribution of such tobacco products to cease.[109] The Secretary's order would affect manufacturers, importers, distributors, and/or retailers.[110] Thus, similar to the Secretary's authority to recall medical devices, the first step of the statute does not require a mandatory recall of the tobacco product for which the Secretary makes the above determination.

As with medical devices, after providing an opportunity for an informal hearing within 10 days of the date the order was issued, the Secretary would be able to amend the order to require recalls of such tobacco products. The Secretary must set a timeline "in which the tobacco product recall will occur."[111] The bills also specify that the Secretary must require reports "describing the progress of the recall," but does not state from whom such reports would be required.[112] Defective tobacco products could not be recalled from individuals, however, an amended order from the Secretary requiring a recall must give notice of the risks associated with using a defective tobacco product. The Secretary could ask retailers and other distributors to notify individuals about the defective tobacco products, which is arguably comparable to the Secretary's ability to use "the assistance of health professionals who prescribed or used" a medical device subjected to a recall.[113]

Again, similar to the Secretary's authority for recalling medical devices, if a significant number of retailers and/or distributors of the defective products cannot be identified,[114] the Secretary must notify these persons by publicizing information under FFDCA § 705(b).[115] Unlike the medical device recall provisions, S. 625 and H.R. 1108 do not provide for replacements, reimbursements, or refunds, however, the bills specify that the value of remedies (potentially, a reimbursement of a retailer's costs associated with replacing the defective products) must be taken into account in an award of damages for economic loss.[116]

End Notes

[1] 21 C.F.R. § 7.3(g). The definition of a recall "does not include a market withdrawal or a stock recovery." *Id.* A market withdrawal is "a firm's removal or correction of a distributed product which involves a minor violation that would not be subject to legal action by the [FDA] or which involves no violation, e.g., normal stock rotation practices, routine equipment adjustments and repairs." 21 C.F.R. § 7.3(j). A stock recovery is "a firm's removal or correction of a product that has not been marketed or that has not left the direct control of the firm, i.e., the product is located on premises owned by, or under the control of, the firm and no portion of the lot has been released for sale or use." 21 C.F.R. § 7.3(k).

[2] More than 1,250 people were sickened in an outbreak linked to jalapeño peppers; 246 deaths of patients receiving heparin were reported to the FDA (though "[i]n the majority of reports with a death outcome, there was not enough clinical information to assess the relationship between death and use of heparin"); and reportedly about "1,950 cats and 2,200 dogs died from kidney failure from eating melamine-contaminated pet food." Annys Shin, *Salmonella-Tainted Jalapeño Found in Texas*, WASH. POST, July 22, 2008, at A1; FDA, Information on Adverse Event Reports and Heparin, [http://www.fda.gov/cder/drug/infopage/heparin/adverse_events.htm]; John Pacenti, *Animal Owners Seek Class Action Status in Suit Over Pet Food Additives*, Law.com, June 10, 2008.

[3] Michael T. Roberts, *Mandatory Recall Authority: A Sensible and Minimalist Approach to Improving Food Safety*, 59:4 FOOD & DRUG L. J. 563, 568 (2004).

[4] Lisa Brennan, *Judge Seethes Over Direct Contact of Represented Parties in Pet Food Case*, N.J. Law Journal, June 4, 2007; Geoff Mulvihill, *Recalled Pet Food Settlement Gets Initial Approval*, Law.com, June 2, 2008.

[5] Katie Zezima, *Tests by Pet Food Maker Killed 7 Animals Before Recall*, N.Y. TIMES, March 20, 2007, at A12.

[6] Chuck Neubauer, *FDA Officials Will Face Senate Inquiry on Pet Food*, LA TIMES, April 8, 2007, at A1 8; *Hearing on Pet Food Safety Before the Senate Subcommittee on Agriculture, Rural Development, Food and Drug Administration, and Related Agencies*, 110th Cong. 6 (April 12, 2007) (statement of Duane Ekedahl, President, Pet Food Institute), [http://appropriations

[7] Center for Science in the Public Interest, *Support H.R. 1612 and S. 908 — The Consumer Food Safety Act of 1999*, [http://www.cspinet.org/foodsafety/hr1612.html]. According to this advocacy organization, "[i]n August 1997, FDA tried to recall Royal Line smoked salmon contaminated with Listeria, a bacteria that causes serious illnesses and deaths. The salmon, sold in plastic packages, was imported from Denmark. However, the salmon's U.S. distributor refused to cooperate in the recall, leaving American consumers at risk of food poisoning from the product." *Id.*

[8] *Veggie Booty Recall Grows, Prompting Criticism of Weak FDA*, Inside Health Policy, July 6, 2007.

[9] *See id.*

[10] "A similar lack of aggressiveness on the part of FDA may have contributed to the peanut butter contamination deaths and illnesses." *Diminished Capacity: Can the FDA Assure the Safety and Security of the Nation's Food Supply — Part 2: Hearing Before the H. Comm. on Energy and Commerce, Subcomm. on Oversight and Investigations*, 110th Cong. (July 17, 2007) (Staff Statement at p. 16), [http://energycommerce.house.gov/cmte_mtgs/110-oi-hrg.071707.Staff-testimony.pdf],(hereinafter "Subcommittee Staff Statement").

[11] Marian Burros, *Who's Watching What We Eat?*, N.Y. Times, May 16, 2007, at D1; R. Robin McDonald, *ConAgra Faces 39 Suits Over Bad Peanut Butter*, Fulton County Daily Report, August 13, 2007. A Centers for Disease Control and Prevention network that monitors food-borne diseases observed a "slowly rising increase" in cases of a certain type of *Salmonella* that were connected to one peanut butter plant. *Id.*

[12] *See* Caroline Smith DeWaal, Director of Food Safety, Center for Science in the Public Interest, Statement at the National Food Policy Conference (May 9, 2003), [http://www. cspinet.org/foodsafety/new_bioact.html].

[13] FDA, Center for Food Safety and Applied Nutrition, Industry Affairs Staff Brochure, *FDA Recall Policies* (June 2002), [http://vm.cfsan.fda.gov/~lrd/recall2.html]. The FDA's recall policies are described in detail in this document.

[14] *Id.*

[15] Ekedahl, *supra* note 6, at 8-9.

[16] *Id.* at 9.

[17] Press Release, Senator Charles Schumer, Schumer Reveals: Chinese Product Dangers Go Far Beyond Tires, Seafood and Toothpaste (July 1, 2007), [http://schumer.senate.gov/SchumerWebsite/pressroom/record.cfm?id=278328]; *see also* FDA, Imported Toothpaste, [http://www.fda.gov/oc/opacom/hottopics/toothpaste.html].

[18] *See Veggie Booty*, *supra* note 8.

[19] GAO, Food Safety: USDA and FDA Need to Better Ensure Prompt and Complete Recalls of Potentially Unsafe Food (October 2004), [http://www.gao.gov/new.items/d055 1 .pdf].

[20] *See id.* at 13-16, 21-22.

[21] Subcommittee Staff Statement, *supra* note 10, at 2.

[22] The U.S. Government does have a single website dedicated to product recalls, [http://www.recalls.gov]. However, this website apparently does not address the concerns of supporters of a single food safety agency, such as two agencies — FDA and USDA — maintaining jurisdiction over eggs in shell, processed, and liquid forms.

[23] In 2004, the FDA found contaminated animal feed but did not report the contamination to the USDA, which inspects livestock that consume such feed, or the state involved, which has authority to prevent such meat from entering the market. The state seized and destroyed the animals before the FDA even sent a warning letter to the feed mill. Government Accountability Office (GAO), Mad Cow Disease: FDA's Management of the Feed Ban Has Improved, but Oversight Weaknesses Continue to Limit Program Effectiveness, 24 (February 2005), [http://www.gao.gov/new.items/d05 101 .pdf].

[24] FDA, Chili Products (Botulism) Recall (Includes Canned Chili, Stew, Hash, BBQ, Gravy, and Pet Food Products), [http://www.fda.gov/oc/opacom/hottopics/castleberry.html#meat

[25] USDA, Food Safety Education, USDA Meat & Poultry Hotline, [http://www.fsis.usda.gov/Food_Safety_Education/USDA_Meat_&_Poultry_Hotline/index.asp]. A press release found after clicking on several links in the USDA website details the chili products with meat that were recalled. Press Release, USDA, Georgia Firm Expands Recall of Canned Meat Products that may Contain *Clostridium botulinum*, [http://www.fsis.usda.gov/ News _& _Events/Recall _033 _2007 _expanded/index. asp].

[26] Timothy M. Hammonds, *It is Time to Designate a Single Food Safety Agency*, 59:3 FOOD & DRUG L. J. 427, 428 (2004); *see, e.g.*, Richard J. Durbin, *Food Safety Oversight for the 21st Century: The Creation of a Single, Independent Federal Food Safety Agency*, 59:3 FOOD & DRUG L. J. 383 (2004); Sandra B. Eskin, *Putting All Your Eggs in One Basket: Egg Safety and the Case for a Single Food-Safety Agency*, 59:3 FOOD & DRUG L. J. 441 (2004).

[27] Stuart M. Pape, Paul D. Rubin, & Heili Kim, *Food Security Would be Compromised by Combining the Food and Drug Administration and the U.S. Department of Agriculture Into a Single Food Agency*, 59:3 FOOD & DRUG L. J. 405, 406 (2004).

[28] *Id.* at 405-06.

[29] *Id.* at 406.

[30] Federal Food, Drug, and Cosmetic Act (FFDCA) § 412(f).

[31] FFDCA § 518(e).

[32] Public Health Service Act § 351; 42 U.S.C. § 262.

[33] FFDCA § 412(f)(1).

[34] FFDCA § 412(f)(2).

[35] 21 C.F.R. § 107.200.

[36] FFDCA § 412(f)(3); *see* 21 C.F.R. § 107.230(d); *see also* 21 C.F.R. § 107.250.

[37] FFDCA § 412(g)(1).

[38] *Id.*

[39] FFDCA § 412(g)(2).

[40] FFDCA § 518(e)(1).

[41] *Id.*

[42] FFDCA § 518(e)(2)(A).

[43] FFDCA § 518(e)(2)(B)(i).

[44] FFDCA § 518(e)(2)(B)(ii).

[45] FFDCA § 518(e)(2)(B).

[46] FFDCA § 705(b).

[47] FFDCA § 5 18(a), (b), (c), (e)(3).

[48] 42 U.S.C. § 262(d)(1); FDA, FDA 101: Biological Products, [http://www.fda.gov/consumer/updates/biologics062608 .html].

[49] 42 U.S.C. § 262(d)(2). The statute provides a formula for adjusting the maximum amount of the civil penalty for violations of the recall statute. *Id.*

[50] 21 C.F.R. §§ 7.1, 7.40.

[51] FDA, FDA REGULATORY PROCEDURES MANUAL, [http://www.fda.gov/ora/compliance ref/rpm].

[52] *See* 21 C.F.R. § 7.40(a).

[53] 21 U.S.C. § 334; FFDCA § 304.

[54] 21 C.F.R. § 7.40(c).

[55] *Id.*

[56] 21 C.F.R. § 7.59.

[57] 21 C.F.R. § 7.46.

[58] *Id.* One example of this may be Menu Foods's expansion of its pet food recall to include cat food varieties. The FDA "had confirmed test results it received from a laboratory . . . [that] found that canned cat food which had not been included in Menu Foods' earlier recalls tested positive for melamine, a chemical used as a fertilizer and in the manufacture of cutlery and kitchenware." The FDA informed Menu Foods, Inc., and the company acted to expand the recall. It is unclear whether the FDA requested the expanded recall or simply informed Menu Foods that the cat food varieties violated the FFDCA. Press Release, FDA, FDA Warns Consumers that Retailers May Still Have Recalled Pet Food on Shelves (April 12, 2007), [http://www.fda.gov/bbs/topics/NEWS/2007/NEW0 1605 .html].

[59] 21 C.F.R. § 7.3(j); *see supra* note 1.

[60] 21 C.F.R. § 7.46(d).

[61] 21 C.F.R. § 7.40(b).

[62] *Id.* The FDA's Associate Commissioner for Regulatory Affairs, who leads the FDA's Office of Regulatory Affairs, "has direct responsibility for approval of all recalls requested by FDA and Class I recalls." Sandra Nowlin Whetstone, *ORA 's Role at FDA Headquarters and in the Field for Product Recalls*, 53:3 FOOD & DRUG L. J. 513, 513 (1998).

[63] 21 C.F.R. § 7.45. When making its request, the FDA notice of the above determinations will state the violation of the FDA-administered laws, the classification of the recall, the recall strategy, and any agency instructions on carrying out the recall. *Id.*

[64] 21 C.F.R. § 7.40(c).

[65] 21 C.F.R. § 7.42(a).

[66] 21 C.F.R. § 7.3(m)(1).

[67] FDA, FDA's Pilot Program to Better Educate Consumers about Recalled Food Products, [http://www.fda.gov/oc/po/firmrecalls/pilot.html].
[68] 21 C.F.R. § 7.3(m)(2) and (3).
[69] FDA, FDA Enforcement Report Index, [http://www.fda.gov/opacom/Enforce.html].
[70] FDA, Recalls, Market Withdrawals and Safety Alerts, [http://www.fda.gov/opacom/ 7alerts.html].
[71] 21 C.F.R. § 7.41(a).
[72] 21 C.F.R. § 7.41.
[73] *Id.* The FDA's Office of Regulatory Affairs' Associate Commissioner "may, and has, delegated designation of certain Class I recalls to the agency's Center directors," such as the Center for Food Safety and Applied Nutrition (CF SAN). Whetstone, *supra* note 62, at 513. "CFSAN's director has been delegated authority for certain routine Class I food recalls, e.g., listeria and undeclared allergen Class I recalls." *Id.*
[74] 21 C.F.R. § 7.49.
[75] 21 C.F.R. § 7.49.
[76] *See supra* note 1.
[77] 21 C.F.R. § 7.50.
[78] 21 C.F.R. § 7.53. The regulations state that "generally the reporting interval will be between 2 and 4 weeks." *Id.*
[79] 21 C.F.R. § 7.53. For example, in the Menu Foods pet food recall, the FDA conducted approximately 400 effectiveness checks in retail stores. *See* Press Release, *supra* note 58.
[80] Whetstone, *supra* note 62, at 514.
[81] 21 C.F.R. § 7.55(a).
[82] *Id.*
[83] Whetstone, *supra* note 62, at 514.
[84] 21 C.F.R. § 7.55(b).
[85] FDA, Regulatory Procedures Manual ch. 7, at 7-25, [http://www.fda.gov/ora/compliance_ref/rpm/pdf/ch7.pdf].
[86] FDA, FDA's Pilot Program to Better Educate Consumers about Recalled Food Products, [http://www.fda.gov/oc/po/firmrecalls/pilot.html].
[87] *Id.*
[88] *Id.* As of July 18, 2007, the FDA received 188 comments. The website states that "[t]he majority of consumers who commented on the pilot find the program beneficial." *Id.*
[89] These provisions were similar to those the Senate approved, by a vote of 94-0, in Senator Durbin's amendment to the FDA Revitalization Act (S. 1082).
[90] P.L. 110-85, § 1003.
[91] P.L. 110-85, § 1002.
[92] P.L. 110-85, § 1002.
[93] S. 1274, § 2; H.R. 2108, § 2 (proposed FFDCA § 417(b)).
[94] S. 1274, § 2; H.R. 2108, § 2 (proposed FFDCA § 4 17(c)).
[95] S. 1274, § 2; H.R. 2108, § 2 (proposed FFDCA § 418(a)(1)).
[96] S. 1274, § 2; H.R. 2108, § 2 (proposed FFDCA § 418(b)).
[97] S. 1274, § 2; H.R. 2108, § 2 (proposed FFDCA § 418(c) and (d)).
[98] S . 1274, § 2; H.R. 2108, § 2 (proposed FFDCA § 418(f)(1)).
[99] S. 1274, § 3; H.R. 2108, § 3.
[100] S. 1274, § 4; H.R. 2108, § 4.
101 The bills define "food establishment" as "a slaughterhouse, factory, warehouse, or facility owned or operated by a person located in any State that processes food or a facility that holds, stores, or transports food or food ingredients." The terms "does not include a farm, restaurant, other retail food establishment, nonprofit food establishment in which food is prepared for or served directly to the consumer, or fishing vessel." S. 654, § 3(13); H.R. 1148, § 3(13).
[102] S. 654, § 205(d); H.R. 1148, § 205(d).
[103] S. 654, § 205(i); H.R. 1148, § 205(i).
[104] S. 654, § 401(11); H.R. 1148, § 401(11).
[105] S. 654, § 405; H.R. 1148, § 405.
[106] H.R. 2099, § 2.
[107] Letter from Wenonah Hauter, Executive Director, Food & Water Watch, to Representative John Dingell, Chairman, House Committee on Energy and Commerce, at 3 (August 17, 2007).
[108] [http://energycommerce.house.gov/FDAGlobalAct-08/Dingel_60AXML.pdf].
[109] S. 625, § 908(c); H.R. 1108, § 908(c).
[110] The medical device recall provisions in the FFDCA call for notification "to health professionals who prescribe or use the device and to any other person (including manufacturers, importers, distributors, retailers, and device users) who should properly receive such notification in order to eliminate such risk." FFDCA § 518(a); 21 U.S.C. § 360h(a).
[111] S. 625, § 908(c)(2)(A); H.R. 1108, § 908(c)(2)(A).

[112] S. 625, § 908(c)(2)(A); H.R. 1108, § 908(c)(2)(A).

[113] FFDCA § 518(e)(2)(B).

[114] S. 625, § 908(c)(2)(B); H.R. 1108, § 908(c)(2)(B).

[115] However, S. 625 and H.R. 1108 do not amend FFDCA § 705(b) to include tobacco products. Section 705(b) currently states that "The Secretary may also cause to be disseminated information regarding *food, drugs, devices, or cosmetics* in situations involving, in the opinion of the Secretary, imminent danger to health or gross deception of the consumer. . . ." (emphasis added).

[116] S . 625, § 908(b); H.R. 1108(b).

In: The Salmonella Outbreak in Peanut Products: The FDA … ISBN: 978-1-60741-950-1
Editor: Benjamin K. Glynn

Chapter 11

OVERSIGHT IN PEANUT RECALL HEARING-DEWAAL (FOOD SAFETY) TESTIMONY

Caroline Smith De Waal

Good morning Mr. Chairman, Ranking Member Chambliss and Members of the Committee. My name is Caroline Smith DeWaal, and I am the director of food safety for the Center for Science in the Public Interest (CSPI). CSPI is a nonprofit health advocacy and education organization focused on food safety, nutrition, and alcohol issues. CSPI is supported principally by the 950,000 subscribers to its *Nutrition Action HealthLetter* and by foundation grants. We accept no government or industry funding.

THE TIME TO REPAIR OUR FOOD SAFETY SYSTEM IS NOW

Thank you for asking me here today to discuss the lessons learned from the latest food-borne disease outbreak linked to peanut products produced by the Peanut Corporation of America (PCA). Let me say that the first lesson we have learned is that the American public cannot wait any longer for solutions to address a seriously broken food safety system.

Over the last two years Congress has conducted seventeen oversight and legislative hearings on food safety that followed outbreaks caused by spinach tainted with *E. coli* O157:H7, peanut butter contaminated with *Salmonella* Tennessee, canned chili sauce with deadly botulism spores, and pet food containing ingredients intentionally adulterated with melamine. In every case, the hearings revealed flaws both in the food manufacturers' processes and in the Food and Drug Administration's oversight. With evidence of both unintentional and intentional contamination leading to large-scale outbreaks, it is little wonder the Government Accountability Office has highlighted the inadequate state of our food regulatory system and placed food safety in its high risk category three years in a row.[1]

Successive outbreaks caused by tainted spinach, lettuce, salad mixes, tomatoes, peppers, pot pies, peanut butter, ground beef, chili sauce, and now numerous products made with contaminated peanuts have demonstrated that our hundred-year-old legal foundation and outdated strategies are inadequate to protect our citizens. Twenty-month-old "CJ" Minto from Mobile, Alabama, contracted *Salmonella* poisoning after eating peanut butter cracker sandwiches that are now part of the recall.[2] CJ's symptoms continued for two weeks, including one week when the child was unable to eat. He was treated with antibiotics for nearly constant diarrhea and vomiting until he resumed eating. Believe it or not, CJ was luckier than some. Shirley Mae Almer was a 72-year old survivor of cancer surgery and radiation therapy. Her family planned to bring her home from a nursing home for Christmas, but she died on December 21 from salmonellosis linked to the peanut butter. A family member said that the death seemed so ironic, "With all the battles she overcame- to have a piece of peanut butter toast take her."[3]

The evidence that FDA reform is needed has been crystal clear in Congressional hearings, victims' stories, and stakeholder agreements. I think you will hear from all the witnesses today that the time for reform is now. Let's begin. And, let's get it right.

Peanut Corporation of America Is the Latest Proof of a Broken Food Safety System

The outbreak of *Salmonella* Typhimirum started in September 2008. The illnesses peaked in December 2008, affecting consumers in 43 states. Though the illnesses have declined since the first announcement on January 10, 2009 that the suspected cause was peanut butter, they have not abated. The *Salmonella* strain has been linked to contaminated products from Peanut Corporation of America. As of January 29, 2009, there have been eight deaths and 550 illnesses linked to PCA's products.[4]

The Peanut Corporation of America supplied peanut butter to nursing homes, schools, hospitals and other institutions, and made peanut paste which became an ingredient in many products. Starting in June 2007, PCA's Blakely, Georgia plant began detecting *Salmonella* in its products and over the next year had 12 occasions when it shipped products that had initially tested positive for *Salmonella*. In each of these 12 separate occasions, instead of addressing the source of the contamination, PCA retested its products to obtain a negative result and then shipped the product.

During this same period, Georgia state inspectors, acting under contract with the FDA, detected a number of violations, but the tests conducted by the state in 2007 failed to detect any contaminants. Georgia inspectors were apparently unaware of the company's own positive tests.

In April 2008, Canada rejected a shipment of peanuts from PCA as unfit for food. PCA attempted to clear the peanuts for sale in the U.S., but FDA rejected its test results and eventually the peanuts were destroyed. FDA did not follow up with an inspection of the plant.

During this period, PCA distributed the contaminated products to more than 100 consignee firms. The peanut paste was used as an ingredient in hundreds of different products, such as cookies, crackers, cereal, candy, and ice cream.

WHAT MUST BE DONE TO REPAIR OUR FOOD SAFETY SYSTEM

The PCA outbreak – like countless episodes in the previous decade – illustrates numerous failures and areas where improvements are needed. The company seemed to have had no food safety operating plan. The company did not respond appropriately to repeated positive *Salmonella* findings. The state of Georgia failed to provide effective inspection, in part because they lacked full access to the plant's food safety records, and FDA failed to provide oversight for the state inspection program. In fact, even when FDA received a clear signal of problems in the plant from its own import alert system, the agency failed to send out inspectors to conduct a review of the plant. Finally, the penalties available to FDA to prosecute the company are not adequate to deter future violations of the Act.

1. Absence of a Food Safety Plan and Response to Positive Test Results

The heart of any effective reform effort lies in prevention, not response. Congress should require every food plant regulated by FDA to have food safety plans detailing that it has analyzed its operations, identified potential hazards, and is taking steps to minimize or prevent contamination. This Hazard Analysis and Critical Control Points (HACCP)-style planning is already a requirement for all meat and poultry plants, and it should be a prerequisite for all food processors that want to sell food in the U.S. This establishes the industry's fundamental responsibility for ensuring food safety and provides a foundation for the government audit inspections. However, the history of these programs in the seafood area demonstrates that Congress must also give FDA the authority and funding to enforce compliance through regular inspections and access to company records.

Additionally, FDA needs the authority to set performance standards for the most hazardous pathogens and to require food processors to meet those standards. The standards are used to ensure that food is produced in a sanitary manner that limits the likelihood of contamination by pathogens, chemicals, or physical hazards, like glass or metal. In the case of PCA, performance standards would have provided inspectors with a benchmark for regular sampling of products.

The approach of HACCP planning combined with performance standards would focus food safety activities on prevention and would permit more efficient and effective government oversight through analysis of records as well as visual and laboratory inspection.

2. The State of Georgia and FDA did not Provide Effective Inspection Oversight

The failures to detect and correct the unsafe practices at PCA highlight how FDA's infrequent inspections (averaging one visit in 10 years)[5] and the agency's oversight of state-contracted inspections contribute to illness outbreaks. FDA hadn't inspected the PCA plant in eight years. Meanwhile, press reports show inspections by the Georgia Department of Agriculture found minor violations that may have pointed to larger problems. It's particularly troubling, though, that the FDA didn't seek either the company's records or the Georgia inspection reports – information that might have prevented the outbreak from occurring - even after it found that some of the products had been rejected by a firm in Canada.

To address these problems, legislation should set specific inspection frequencies for all food plants. Higher-risk foods should be inspected at a greater frequency, preferably no less than annually, with lower risk food facilities being inspected at least once in any two year period. Those inspection rates would still be well below the rate established for restaurant inspections of once every six months.[6] Setting frequencies will require a commitment to fund the agency or find new resources, and some legislative proposals have established a modest registration fee to offset the costs associated with increased inspection oversight. Current FDA funding shortfalls have reached a critical level, leaving the agency with fewer inspectors, even as the workload continues to increase. Since 1972, domestic inspections conducted by FDA declined 81 percent.[7] Just since 2003, the number of FDA field staff dropped by 12 percent, and between 2003 and 2006, there was a 47 percent drop in federal inspections.[8] Just those declines in inspectors and inspections can be traced to an ongoing funding shortfall in the food safety program estimated in the hundreds of millions of dollars.[9]

FDA and state inspectors are also hampered in conducting inspections by restricted access to plant records that could have identified problems at PCA. After the outbreak, FDA obtained records of 12 tests that were positive for *Salmonella* in the year leading up to the outbreak that had not been disclosed to inspectors. PCA was within its rights under current law to refuse to disclose the tests even if asked by inspectors in the plant. This is because inspectors cannot access records unless the requirements of the Bioterrorism Act are met and the inspector presents a written demand.[10] We saw this same situation play out in the 2007 Peter Pan peanut butter outbreak where, had inspectors been given access to test records, they would have been alerted to test the plant for *Salmonella*.[11] Even after the PCA outbreak was ongoing, the FDA had to invoke the Bioterrorism Act to access PCA's records. This is unacceptable. To fix this, the law needs to be changed so that inspectors during routine inspections have access to the results of tests conducted by the plant. The ability to access plant food safety records during inspections is an essential tool to identifying problems. As it turned out, PCA , instead of fixing the problem, fixed the tests, something FDA could have determined had it been given access to the records.

With regard to the shortcomings in state inspection, we must avoid drawing the wrong conclusions. Instead of illustrating that Federal/State cooperation is unreliable, the PCA example argues for improving federal oversight of and assistance to state inspectors who are used to leverage resources for inspections.

In addition to leveraging inspection resources, state health departments are the front line for detecting outbreaks. The Minnesota Department of Health with its innovative approach to epidemiology determined that peanut products were the source of the outbreak. Yet, many states do not have the resources to establish programs modeled on Minnesota's. Congress needs to strengthen the state inspection and surveillance system by providing assistance through training and grants.

While federal and state inspections and surveillance can be improved, they will never be perfect. Congress also should consider leveraging concerned citizens as a means of detecting and preventing situations that can lead to outbreaks. We should protect responsible citizens who come forward to reveal hazards that could affect public health. Whistleblower protections would prevent bureaucratic and corporate hazing of workers to prevent them from coming forward with information about misconduct. We cannot know whether a concerned worker may have come forward in the case of PCA to reveal the positive tests had he or she been protected from retaliation. But all necessary tools to prevent a similar outbreak should be considered.

3. FDA does not Have Effective Penalties for PCA and for Deterring Similar Actions by Other Companies

The punishment for committing a prohibited act under the Food, Drug and Cosmetic Act is up to a year in jail, a $1,000 fine or both.[12] This punishment, which may have been substantial in 1938, has not kept pace with the modern commercial world. Compared to PCA's annual revenues of $17.5 million[13] it is hard to see how a misdemeanor fine serves as an incentive for companies to improve their food safety practices. With over 500 people reported sick, more than 100 hospitalized and eight dead as a result of PCA putting contaminated product on the market, such trivial fines – even if found for numerous violations – do not appear fair.

Criminal liability is also a burden on the agency inspectors, as it must conduct a criminal investigation, coordinate prosecution with the Justice Department, and then go through a criminal trial to recover a fairly modest fine or sentence a culpable individual to a misdemeanor jail term.[14] Another approach Congress should consider is to provide the agency with authority to impose substantial civil penalties that can get the attention of managers and be sustained if violations are continuous. Civil liability provides a flexible deterrent to corporate misconduct that can be tailored to the violation. These remedies are available for addressing violations on the drug and device side of FDA, but not the food side except for illegal pesticide residue.[15] It is time to bring FDA's penalties for food violations in line with what is used for drugs and medical devices.

4. FDA does not Require Effective Traceability Systems, and Lacks Adequate Authority to Protect Consumers by Detaining and Ordering Recalls of Unsafe Food

The ability to trace products and their ingredients is essential to speeding up response when an outbreak occurs. Under the Bioterrorism Act, food companies must maintain a record of the immediate previous source and the immediate subsequent recipient of food.[16] The effort to identify the source of the PCA outbreak illustrates areas where traceback could be improved.

The process of determining the source of an outbreak is difficult and time consuming. The Minnesota Department of Health has one of the best epidemiology programs in the country. Faced with nine reports of *Salmonella* poisoning in the State, the department began interviewing victims and comparing data to find a source. The interviews turned up peanut butter, but because PCA provided ingredients to many manufacturers, the epidemiologists could not identify a single brand. As one investigator said, "We had a lot of peanut butter eaters, but none of the brand names were matching up well."[17] A traceability systems that requires processors to recorded the sources of ingredients and provide those records to investigators could have turned up the correlation between the various brands and their single supplier, PCA.

While all of the companies involved in the peanut recall have acted responsibly, CSPI continues to believe that giving FDA authority to order a recall if necessary is a critical tool for responding to future outbreaks. Today, when you see the notices of the recall, they often mention that it is voluntary. Unfortunately, while true, this may not compel consumers to act with urgency, because they might reason "If it were serious, FDA would issue a mandatory recall."

Conclusion

President Barack Obama has promised a "government that works," and recently promised a complete review of the FDA's food safety program. Luckily for the President and the public, Congress has been investigating problems at the FDA for several years, and many elements of a reform plan are "shovel ready" – they could be accomplished quickly and deliver real benefits to consumers.

But to deal with the root of the problem, Congress and the Obama Administration will need to go beyond giving the FDA more authority and funding. Structural reforms are also essential. Although the FDA is responsible for the safety of 80 percent of the food supply, the FDA's commissioner must divide his or her attention among drugs, medical devices, foods and cosmetics – and food issues frequently fall to the bottom of the pile. Food responsibilities are divided among at least three centers within the FDA, and there is no single food safety expert in charge of the policies, budget and enforcement staff. This means there is no credible voice communicating to the public and the industry what can be done to prevent outbreaks.

It is time to elevate the food monitoring function within the Department of Health and Human Services, which oversees the FDA. The agency needs to be divided in two, with a new Commissioner of Food and Nutrition Policy who reports directly to the HHS Secretary. Food safety functions under the Department of Agriculture have this sort of direct reporting, leading to greater involvement by the Secretary of Agriculture when problems arise in the meat area.

Now is the time for Congress to fundamentally reform and fully fund our food safety system. Enactment by the end of this year should be the goal. Two years ago, Congress expressed its commitment to adopt a modern regulatory oversight program and fund it adequately to fulfill its mission in the Food and Drug Administration Amendments Act of 2007.[18] Bipartisan legislation introduced in the Senate in the last term of Congress further demonstrated readiness to address problems with FDA's food program. That bipartisanship emerged at the same time coalitions of traditionally estranged consumer and industry organizations, like the Alliance for a Stronger FDA, are appealing to many in Congress to rebuild the agency. With both the public and the regulated industries clamoring for change there is no reason to delay. Preventing future illnesses and deaths – future CJs and Shirley Maes – is within our grasp.

End Notes

[1] Gov. Acct. Off., *High Risk Update: Revamping Federal Oversight of Food Safety*, Rep. No. GAO-09-271, Jan. 2009.

[2] Jane Akre, Salmonella Victim Speaks Out, Injuryboard.com, Jan. 30, 2009, at http://www.injuryboard.com/national-news/salmonella

[3] David Shaffer, *Heartbreak Lawsuit; The Family of a Perham, Minn., Woman Who Died of a Salmonella Infection is Suing a Peanut Butter Manufacturer and Asking for Safer Food*, Minn. Star Tribute, Jan. 27, 2009.

[4] Centers for Disease Control, *Investigation Update: Outbreak of Salmonella Typhimurium Infections, 2008–2009*, (accessed Feb. 3, 2009) at http://www.cdc.gov/salmonella

[5] House Comm. on Gov't Reform, *Fact Sheet: Weaknesses in FDA's Food Safety System*, (Oct. 30, 2006), *at* http://oversight

[6] Center for Science in the Public Interest, *Dirty Dining: Have Reservations? You Will Now.*, 2008, at http://cspinet.org/new/pdf/ddreport.pdf.

[7] *Id.*

[8] Andrew Bridges & Seth Borenstein, *AP Investigation: Food Safety Inspections Lanquish*, Associated Press, Feb. 29, 2007, at http://abcnews.go.com/Health/wireStory?id

[9] FDA Science Board Subcommittee on Technology, *FDA's Mission at Risk: Estimated Resources Required for Implementation*. Feb. 25, 2008.

[10] 21 U.S.C. § 374(a)(1)(B); FDA, Regulatory Procedures Manual 2008, § 10-4-3.

[11] Two years before the outbreak, the plant manager refused an oral request from FDA inspectors to see company records of a positive Salmonella test telling them they would need a written request. Marion Burros, *Who's Watching What We Eat*, N.Y. Times, May 16, 2007, at http://www.nytimes.com/2007/05/16/dining/16fda.html.

[12] 21 U.S.C. § 333(a)(1).

[13] Peanut Corporation of America Company Profile, Bizjournals.com, (accessed Feb. 3, 2009), *at* http://www.bizjournals.com/gen/company.html?gcode=904819E282CB4C8B9DAE476F9A3F632D.

[14] For a description of FDA's procedures for prosecuting a case see section 6-5 of the Regulatory Procedures Manual, supra, note 9.

[15] Civil penalties for pesticide residue are found at 21 U.S.C. § 333(f)(2).

[16] 21 U.S.C. § 350c(b).

[17] Gardiner Harris & Pam Belluck, *New Look at Food Safety After Peanut Tainting*, NY Times, Jan. 3,0, 2009.

[18] Food and Drug Administration Amendments Act of 2007, Pub. L. 110-85 § 1005, 121 Stat. 823, (2007).

In: The Salmonella Outbreak in Peanut Products: The FDA … ISBN: 978-1-60741-950-1
Editor: Benjamin K. Glynn

Chapter 12

OVERSIGHT IN PEANUT RECALL HEARING-HUBBARD TESTIMONY

William K. Hubbard

INTRODUCTION

Mr. Chairman and members of the Committee, I am William K. Hubbard. Before my retirement after 33 years of Federal service, I served for many years with the U.S. Food and Drug Administration, and for my last 14 years was an FDA Associate Commissioner responsible for, among other things, FDA's regulations and policy development. Today, I serve as an advisor to The Alliance for a Stronger FDA, a consortium of patient, public interest, and industry organizations whose mission is to urge that FDA's appropriations be increased. The Alliance and its constituent members are greatly concerned that FDA's resource limitations have hampered the agency's ability to ensure the safety of our food and drug supply. Today's hearing is focused on the recent salmonella outbreak that been so costly to the public, and on what directions our food regulatory system might go to prevent further such outbreaks. I commend the Committee for your effort to shine light on this problem and possible solutions.

BACKGROUND

As you know, Congress established the Food and Drug Administration in 1906 as a result of concerns about the safety of our food supply. In those days, it was common for foods to be subjected to all manner of problematic practices—filthy, unsanitary conditions were common in food processing facilities; talcum powder, sawdust and many other contaminants were added to deceptively increase the weight or value of foods; and chemical preservatives were used in food that were untested and often highly toxic. As the 20th Century progressed, FDA's scientists and those in the emerging food processing industry slowly built a food safety infrastructure for the United States that enabled us to claim that we had the safest food supply in the world. And the standards established by the FDA for the production of safe foods became the model for protection around the globe. Throughout the last century, there was steady progress in the food safety system – in learning how to protect food from contamination and in implementing procedures to translate that knowledge into safer food production. But, unfortunately, that record of progress appears to have largely ground to a halt, at least when it comes to the ability of FDA to effectively oversee improvements in food safety, and the limitations under which FDA attempts to do its job have been dismayingly exposed.

And that slowdown in FDA's role –some would even say reversal – has come at the worst possible time. That is because today the need for effective management of food safety is greater than ever before, as evidenced by:

The emergence of new pathogens, some unknown to science in years past, such as E Coli 0157:H7, that are especially lethal when they contaminate our food;

The substantial public health and economic costs imposed on our society from the steady – and increasing – numbers of foodborne disease outbreaks in the United States;

The steady growth in the number of domestic food producers and, even more importantly, the tremendous increase of imported food from other countries—particularly developing countries in Latin America and Asia, where food safety standards are often lax or unenforced; and

The increasing complexity of our system of food production and distribution, which often necessitates the movement of food across long distances and through many hands and into many finished products.

THE SALMONELLA IN PEANUT BUTTER OUTBREAK

The occasion for this hearing is, of course, the recent (and perhaps ongoing) series of cases of Salmonella Typhimurium linked to peanut butter. With hundreds of illnesses, and several deaths, reported, and many more likely not documented; the recall of a wide variety of food products made by many different producers; and widespread consumer anxiety about a food commonly consumed by our children, including our new President's daughter, it is a significant event in our national life.

The questions raised by this outbreak are numerous:

1. Is the Federal government properly organized to manage an outbreak of this nature?
2. Are the various governmental entities involved in foodborne disease outbreaks – Federal, state, and local – adequately coordinated?
3. Does FDA have the necessary authorities and resources to prevent such contaminations and outbreaks from continuing?
4. Are state food inspectors properly trained and managed to insure effective partnership with Federal food safety efforts?
5. Are FDA and industry processes for tracing the source and destination of food products adequate to ensure rapid recall of contaminated food?

I suggest, Mr. Chairman, that we, as a nation, have not demonstrated that we take the threat to our food supply seriously. We talk a great deal about the need to improve food safety, and wring our hands over each major outbreak that occurs, costing lives and industry resources. But our actions have not been consistent with our rhetoric. Let me explain.

TOLL OF FOODBORNE ILLNESS

As you know, the Centers for Disease Control estimate that 76 million Americans contract a foodborne illness each year. Of those, 350,000 are hospitalized, and 5,000 die. That means that we are losing the equivalent of the World Trade Center attack every 8 months, yet many, if not most, of those deaths are preventable. And beyond the obvious human suffering, and the associated economic costs to sickened consumers, there are tremendous economic costs to food producers. The 2006 spinach outbreak, for example, resulted in the destruction of much of that year's spinach crop and cost producers an estimated $100 million; and last year's tomato/pepper outbreak resulted in producer losses in the hundreds of million of dollars. In fact, it is estimated that the overall negative economic impact of foodborne illness in the United States may be has high as $83 billion per year. Worse yet, these repeated outbreaks and their attendant publicity paint a picture, erroneously I believe, of a food industry that cannot assure safe products. Indeed, after the spinach outbreak, the government of Mexico – a nation derided in the past as the home of Montezuma's Revenge – announced it would evaluate whether American produce was safe to import into Mexico. And this is happening at a time in which one of America's few remaining sources of a positive trade balance is our food exports.

FDA'S FOOD SAFETY SYSTEM – BROKEN BEYOND REPAIR?

"FDA does not have the capacity to ensure the safety of food for the nation." Those are not my words, but rather the summation last year of FDA's Science Board, an advisory committee of experts from many fields of study. And that conclusion has been echoed by a cascade of expert reports in recent years, by the Institute of Medicine, the Government Accountability Office, the HHS Inspector General, the National Academies of Science, and several Congressional committees. All of those studies have concluded that the FDA regulatory system, as currently constructed, simply cannot adequately oversee a large and diverse food production system within its current structure and resources.

Let me give you just a flavor of the metrics by which FDA's inability can be counted. When I arrived at FDA in the 1970s, the Official Establishment Inventory of food facilities subject to regulation was about 70,000, and FDA was able to inspect each of those facilities every other year (that is, 35,000 inspections per year). Today, the OEI is 150,000, and FDA conducts about 7,000 inspections per year. This means that FDA can realistically inspect only the 6,000 or so facilities that are designated as "high risk," meaning that most food facilities never see an FDA inspector. [Peanut butter has not been considered a high risk food.] Attached is a chart illustrating the dramatic decline in food inspections since the 1970s.

This also means that in the days when FDA's food program was adequately resourced, FDA would have likely inspected the Blakely, Georgia peanut butter processor with some regularity, but today the chances of FDA routinely visiting that facility are virtually nil. And, of course, it further means that there could be, and likely are, many other facilities around the country with similar problems awaiting their turn in the limelight.

The more recent history of FDA capacity is even more disheartening. In 2003, FDA had just over 4000 field investigators and compliance officers to inspect our food facilities and track down problems like the current salmonella outbreak (as well as inspect drug and medical device facilities). Entering 2008, that force had been reduced to 3354, a loss of almost 700 inspectors. The cadre of food scientists in FDA headquarters underwent a 20% reduction during that time (from 950 to 782). And this occurred as the number of foodborne disease outbreaks more than doubled. These recent trends are part of a larger scenario over many years, in which we have declined to provide the FDA with robust capacity to oversee the safety of our food. And, of course, none of this counts the 216,000 foreign facilities making food for our market, of which FDA inspects only about 100 per year.

An Ineffective Paradigm

I will not dwell on FDA's resource woes; they have been well documented and are indisputable. The more important point is that the resource shortfalls are secondary to the real problem, which is that FDA's food safety system is a relic of the 19th century, one that should have been discarded years ago.

Let's look back to FDA's origins, in the dawn of the 20th century. Americans grew much of their food, and food that was purchased tended to come from a nearby source, such as a farm near the consumer's home. Processed foods were relatively few in number, and tended to be staple goods, such as molasses, flour, and sugar. Some of the most lethal bacterial "pathogens" that worry us today, such as E Coli 0157:H7, were unknown to nature and thus no threat to humans. The "state of the art" method of ensuring food safety was the visual inspection by a government official of food processing facilities and the products emanating from them. Imports were few, and were also mostly staple goods. An inspector could easily open a barrel of flour and examine it for insect or rodent infestation, mold and mildew, and other signs of contamination. So Congress embodied that concept into the original Pure Food and Drug Act. Itinerant Federal inspectors could visit facilities and examine their overall sanitation as an indicator of safe food production. With new provisions added in 1938, those inspectors were give enforcement tools believed to be adequate for the day – prosecution of the business's chief executive, an injunction against the business to stop it from selling contaminated food, and authority to seize food found to be contaminated.

Meat, on the other hand, was considered a far riskier food in those pre-refrigeration days. That concern, combined with the need to assure export markets that U.S. beef was free of brucellosis and hoof and mouth disease, prompted Congress to require a continuous inspection model for slaughter facilities, in which Federal inspectors examine and provide a Federal stamp to every meat product as it is processed; that system remains largely unchanged today.

While the meat inspection program also has its critics, the FDA food safety system has been determined to have severe flaws in its conception and implementation, in the context of the modern world, viz.,

It is a system with random success. That is, it relies on the infrequent inspection by FDA (or perhaps a state inspector) to identify and correct deficiencies in a processing facility;

Each FDA inspection is only a "snapshot" of the condition of the food processor the day of the visit, thus it cannot assure that the facility is operating safely at all times;

There are few true standards by which most food processors can be judged. FDA has general "sanitation" regulations, but has not been empowered to set food- specific requirements to which producers should adhere;

It does not take advantage of state-of-the-art food protection mechanisms (e.g., HACCP) that industry leaders have developed and implemented in recent years;

Food safety inspections and oversight by state and local authorities are inadequately coordinated with the FDA; nor are training of state and local inspectors done jointly with FDA inspectors, resulting in differing inspection procedures and varying thoroughness;

It lacks enforcement tools common to modern regulatory agencies, such as authority to recall contaminated food, to require periodic registration of food facilities, to fine firms failing to comply with requirements, and to require detailed records of a food's movement through commerce (so that contaminated food can be found and recalled promptly); and

FDA lacks a modern and robust laboratory system that can effectively and rapidly test food samples for the hundreds of possible contaminants that can attack our food.

What is Needed – A Modern, Risk-Based Food Safety System

Despite the considerable gloom we have been seeing in recent years related to the failures of our food safety system, there is great reason to be optimistic that we can successfully fix its many flaws. The key will be to move from the current reactive, fragmented system to one that is focused on prevention. FDA and the industry have already demonstrated the possibilities, through development of procedures for preventive controls for low-acid canned foods, seafood, and juice. Known generally as Hazard Analysis Critical Control Points, or HACCP, it is a methodology under which producers undertake four steps to assure the safety of their food, and whose complexity is based on the risks posed to the food:

1. *Analyze hazards*, that is, understand what hazards their food might be subjected to so that they can eliminate them,
2. *Develop a food safety plan* under which they will take the necessary steps to control the identified hazards,
3. *Document the steps* the facility takes to implement the plan, thereby creating a record of how they successfully control the hazards, and can thus assure both regulators and their customers that they are always vigilant about food safety, and

4. *Meet standards* for minimizing risk in their food, such as by periodic testing for hazards to assure that the finished product is indeed uncontaminated.

These are often fairly simple, common sense steps, but they have shown a remarkable capacity to effectively prevent food contamination. In the case of a peanut butter processor, for example, the four steps might be implemented as follows:

1. *Hazard identification* would likely be focused on bacterial contamination,
2. *The food safety plan* would identify the need to a) roast the raw peanuts at sufficiently high temperature to ensure that any bacteria arriving from the farm is killed, then, b) keep the processing equipment clean so that the peanut butter is not exposed to bacteria while being processed and packaged. This would also include the need to guard against rodent and insect infestation, leaky roofs, and any other threat to equipment sanitation.
3. *Documentation* might include only temperature recording of the roaster while it is in operation and the recording of regular, thorough cleaning of the processing equipment; and, finally,
4. Performance *Standards* could be met by periodic sampling and testing of the final product, to confirm that it is free of bacteria.

Under such a new paradigm, FDA's role would shift from its current "gotcha" mode via random inspections to one in which they set the requirements for preventive controls and any necessary quantitative tolerances for contaminants, train and educate processors in the use of such controls, assess the adequacy of firms' food safety plans, and oversee an inspection regime under which FDA, state, local, and other third-party inspectors can confirm the proper implementation of food safety plans.

WHAT IS NEEDED FROM CONGRESS

FDA cannot move to the type of modern food safety system that is needed without statutory change. Specifically, I believe the Congress should enact legislation with the following elements:

First, *empower FDA to mandate preventive controls for all food.* Many, if not most, large processors have already adopted some form of preventive controls, but such a system will only be as strong as its weakest link, and FDA must be specifically charged with requiring universal HACCP-like processes.

Second, *give FDA the resources to be successful in a new food safety system.* In the 1970s, when FDA's food program was at its zenith, its budget was one-half of the agency's budget, and that could be a goal for restoring the program to health. It would require additional funding of about $500 million, or about 2 cents a week for each American. Without the resources to strengthen the FDA, no authorities can or will bring the change that is needed, but I believe the vast majority of Americans would gladly pay a penny every few days for a safer food supply. Indeed, the cost to the taxpayer would likely be recouped by savings to consumers through the elimination of just one major outbreak a year.

Third, enact long overdue *enforcement authorities* for FDA, such as mandatory recall authority, annual registration for all food facilities, a revised administrative detention authority, accreditation of private laboratories, and a stronger traceback authority. Fourth, direct the Secretary of Health and Human Services to develop an effective *crisis management system* that coordinates the response to foodborne disease outbreaks among CDC, FDA, and state and local government; cuts through the current bickering and turf battles among those entities; and effectively shortens the response time and resolution of future outbreak.

And, fifth, authorize and fund a *food safety training academy* that will provide uniform, science-based training for all food inspectors, at all levels of government and in the private sector.

A NEED TO MOVE FROM TALK TO ACTION

In conclusion, Mr. Chairman, today's hearing is another in a series that Congress has held to highlight instances where FDA needs to improve, and I agree with your concerns that FDA is not as effective as it can and should be. In the case of food, we have a real dichotomy between our rhetoric and our action. As I noted earlier, we say we want a strong FDA and a strong food safety system, but our actions belie that stated objective. We have not given FDA the authority and resources it needs to be the agency we want it to be, and then we are critical of it when it fails to meet expectations. Meanwhile, as report after report recommends dramatic change in our food safety oversight, the number of foodborne disease outbreaks have risen from about 100 per year fifteen years ago to 350 per year more recently. That is a record for which we should be truly embarrassed, and I sincerely hope that you and your colleagues will agree with my conclusions and resolve to act upon them.

Thank you for giving me the opportunity to provide my views on this subject.

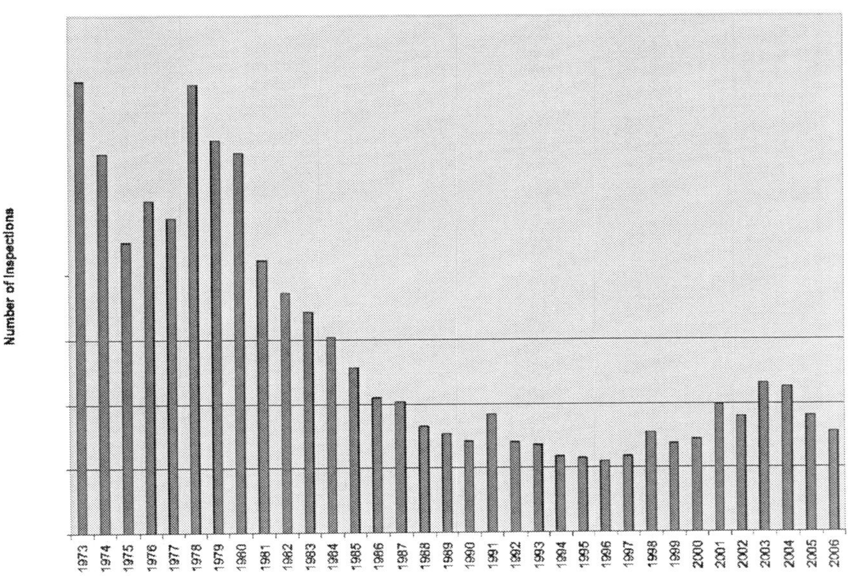

Food Inspections 1973-2006

In: The Salmonella Outbreak in Peanut Products: The FDA ... ISBN: 978-1-60741-950-1
Editor: Benjamin K. Glynn

Chapter 13

Oversight in Peanut Recall Hearing-Khan (CDC) Testimony

Ali Khan

Introduction

Good morning, Chairman Harkin and Members of the Committee. I am Ali Khan, an Assistant Surgeon General and Deputy Director of the National Center for Zoonotic, Vector-Borne, and Enteric Diseases, at the Centers for Disease Control and Prevention (CDC). Thank you for the invitation to address the Committee on CDC's activities related to the prevention of foodborne disease and CDC's role in the response to the current outbreak of *Salmonella* Typhimurium infections associated with peanut containing products.

Background

Diseases spread by contaminated foods continue to challenge the public health system. Large foodborne outbreaks now often are attributed to fresh produce and processed foods, as well as foods of animal origin. Numerous factors are responsible for these large outbreaks such as the complexity of evolving microbes and changing food consumption patterns. In addition, CDC relies on local and state health departments, which have varying capacity to detect and respond to food-related illnesses

As an agency within the Department of Health and Human Services (HHS), CDC leads federal efforts to gather data on foodborne illnesses, investigate foodborne illnesses and outbreaks, and monitor the effectiveness of prevention and control efforts. CDC is not a food safety regulatory agency, but CDC works closely with the food safety regulatory agencies, in particular with HHS's Food and Drug Administration (FDA) and the Food Safety and Inspection Service within the United States Department of Agriculture (USDA/FSIS). CDC also plays a key role in building state and local health department epidemiology, laboratory, environmental health, and communication capacity to support foodborne disease surveillance and outbreak response. Importantly, CDC data can be used to help document the effectiveness of prevention interventions.

Everything that CDC does depends on critical partnerships with state and local public health departments that collect surveillance data, conduct laboratory testing, investigate most outbreaks, and take public health action. CDC has worked with the Association of Public Health Laboratories (APHL) and the Council of State and Territorial Epidemiologists (CSTE) to develop networks for foodborne disease surveillance. For example, PulseNet, the national network for molecular subtyping of foodborne bacteria coordinated by CDC, allows every state health laboratory to test strains of bacteria from sick persons in that state and to compare them with DNA "fingerprint" patterns in the national database at CDC. This has greatly improved the ability to detect clusters of illness that may be related, even if they are dispersed across multiple states. There are similarly other related systems that coordinate the investigation of the large, multistate clusters detected by PulseNet [OutbreakNet team], facilitate state reporting of outbreaks to CDC [National Outbreak Reporting System], develop baseline information on what foods are commonly consumed and trends in foodborne illness [FoodNet], and assess policies and practices of retail foodservice establishments that could lead to or prevent foodborne outbreaks [Environmental Health Specialist Network].

CDC also works with a broad range of other partners to improve capacity and knowledge regarding foodborne disease control and prevention. In collaboration with the National Environmental Health Association (NEHA), CDC conducts team training programs for local and state health department officials including specialists in environmental health, laboratory science, and epidemiology. CDC works with the World Health Organization (WHO) and a variety of other international partners to conduct similar training programs in other countries. CDC supports the Council to Improve Foodborne Outbreak Response (CIFOR), which was created to help develop model programs and processes that will facilitate the investigation and control of foodborne disease outbreaks. CSTE and the National Association of County and City Health Officials (NACCHO) are co-chairing CIFOR, and it includes representatives from CDC, FDA, USDA, APHL, NEHA, the Association of State and Territorial Health Officials, the Association of Food and Drug Officials, and industry.

SALMONELLA

Salmonella is a group of bacteria that is widespread in the intestines of birds, reptiles, and mammals. *Salmonella* is the most commonly diagnosed bacterial cause of foodborne diseases in the U.S., causing 15 reported laboratory-confirmed infections per 100,000 persons in 2007, as measured in FoodNet. There are many different kinds, or serotypes, of *Salmonella* bacteria. Serotyping is a classification system based on differences in structures on the surfaces of bacteria or other disease-causing agents. Serotyping performed by public health laboratories around the nation divides *Salmonella* into more than 2,500 different serotypes, some common and some rare. Serotype Typhimurium is the most common serotype in the U.S. and causes 15-20 outbreaks every year. In 2006, Typhimurium represented 19% of reported *Salmonella* illnesses. Each serotype can be further sub-divided into many more subtypes based on additional laboratory tests of their DNA.

Salmonella infections have often been associated with meat, poultry, eggs, and raw milk; these products are derived from animals that can carry *Salmonella*. *Salmonella* has also been associated with fresh produce and other plant-derived foods and can be transmitted through processed foods, like pot pies, breakfast cereal, snack foods, and peanut butter. *Salmonella*, like other pathogens that are commonly foodborne, can also be transmitted in other ways besides food, such as from contact with reptiles or other animals, between children at a child care center, or in water.

Many foodborne infections, including *Salmonella*, occur in persons without obvious connections to each other. These are called sporadic cases; determining the source of a single sporadic case can be very difficult. Cases of similar infections can also occur as a group or "cluster." Epidemiological investigation of clusters of possibly related cases permits public health officials to determine if the cases were connected and, specifically, if they were linked to food. A cluster of foodborne illnesses is considered an outbreak if an investigation demonstrates that two or more infections caused by the same agent are linked to the same food.

In general, for a foodborne illness to be recognized by the public health surveillance system, a patient must seek medical attention; the physician must decide to order diagnostic tests; and the laboratory must conduct the test using the appropriate procedures and report the results to a health department. Many ill people do not seek medical attention, and of those who do, many are not tested for *Salmonella* or other agents causing food borne illness. Therefore, many cases of foodborne illness are neither diagnosed nor reported. For example, *Salmonella* infection has been estimated to cause about 1.4 million foodborne illnesses annually; however, only about 40,000 laboratory-confirmed cases of *Salmonella* are reported to CDC each year.

Regular reporting about detection of *Salmonella* serotypes and subtypes from ill persons is critical in determining whether a surge in incidence has occurred signaling a possible outbreak. Each serotype can be further divided by DNA analysis into subtypes that are distinguished by different DNA fingerprint patterns. The fingerprint pattern is determined with a test known as pulsed-field gel electrophoresis (PFGE). PFGE is a very good method for differentiating among epidemiologically unrelated isolates of many serotypes.

Public health laboratories determine the serotype and PFGE patterns for *Salmonella* strains and share the patterns through PulseNet. The laboratories participating in PulseNet are in state health departments, some local health departments, USDA, and FDA. When a clinical laboratory detects *Salmonella* from an ill person, a sample is sent to a State or local PulseNet laboratory where it is serotyped and DNA fingerprinted. The laboratory compares the fingerprint pattern to that of other *Salmonella* strains from people in that area and uploads the pattern electronically to the national PulseNet database maintained at CDC, where it can be compared with patterns from all over the country. This gives us the capability to detect an unusual number of *Salmonella* cases with the same pattern in a single area or in multiple states. The system can identify patterns even if the affected persons live far apart, which is important given the widespread U.S. food distribution systems. Thousands of different fingerprints have been described, and it is not unusual to find some matches in the system, and at any given moment, the PulseNet system may be tracking many small clusters. When the number of matching strains in a cluster increases, and the number of states reporting the matching pattern increases, then the cluster is flagged for investigation at the national level.

The current outbreak is caused by *Salmonella* with two closely related patterns that had not been seen in PulseNet before this outbreak.

The current outbreak represents a typical timeline for detecting and investigating foodborne illnesses. There is an inherent time lapse between when a person becomes ill with *Salmonella* infection and when the results of testing are reported to PulseNet. It takes time for a person to become ill, seek medical care, and submit a sample for testing. It then takes time for the clinical laboratory to detect *Salmonella* and send the strain to the public health laboratory; finally, the public health laboratory must perform serotyping and DNA fingerprinting and then submit that finding to Pulsenet, which is when CDC becomes aware of the illness.

The Current Salmonella Typhimurium Outbreak

On November 10, 2008, CDC's PulseNet staff noted a small and highly dispersed multistate cluster of 13 *S.* Typhimurium isolates with an unusual PFGE pattern reported from 12 states, and the OutbreakNet team began monitoring it. On November 25, CDC worked with state and local partners to begin an epidemiologic assessment of that cluster, which had increased to 35 isolates reported from 16 states. On December 2, CDC and state and local partners began an assessment of a second cluster of 41 *S.* Typhimurium isolates from 17 states. The PFGE patterns of the second cluster were very similar to the patterns in the first cluster. This second cluster had been first noted by PulseNet on November 24, as a cluster of 27 isolates from 14 states. Neither of these patterns was seen previously in the PulseNet *S.* Typhimurium database. In December, the two clusters were being investigated in parallel because they appeared to be similar. On January 7, 2009, after *Salmonella* from the two patterns were shown to be indistinguishable by other advanced laboratory tests, the two patterns were grouped together as a single outbreak strain, and the investigations were merged.

The initial steps in an epidemiological investigation are to collect information from which hypotheses can be generated about the possible source of the outbreak. As cases with the same DNA fingerprint pattern were identified, CDC collaborated with public health professionals in local and state health departments who were interviewing patients to determine what specific foods or other exposures they may have had in common. Many affected state and local health departments, including the Minnesota Department of Health (MDH), conducted intensive investigations of patients infected with the outbreak strain and shared the findings with CDC. These interviews did not immediately point to a specific product, but raised the possibility of peanut butter and chicken products, without suggesting a particular brand.

By December 28, the Minnesota Department of Health had learned from patient interviews that some patients infected with the outbreak strain lived or ate meals in one of at least three institutions (two long-term care facilities and one elementary school). A review of menus and invoices by MDH and the Minnesota Department of Agriculture (MDA) revealed that the institutions had a common food distributor in North Dakota, and the only food common to the three institutions was King Nut creamy peanut butter. By January 9, 2009, six additional cases in six other Minnesota institutions were identified by MDH; each of those institutions had received King Nut peanut butter. On January 9, the MDA laboratory reported isolation of *Salmonella* from an open container of King Nut peanut butter. This was confirmed on January 12 as *S*. Typhimurium of the outbreak strain.

On January 3 and 4, 2009, data were gathered for a study by CDC and state and local health departments to identify whether illness was associated with eating specific food items. Preliminary analysis found that ill persons were significantly more likely than non-ill persons to have eaten peanut butter, though illness was not associated with eating national brands of jarred peanut butter sold in grocery stores. By January 9, when an opened jar of King Nut peanut butter collected at a nursing home in Minnesota was reported to be growing an as yet uncharacterized *Salmonella*, the FDA had identified a Peanut Corporation of America (PCA) factory in Blakely, Georgia, as the sole producer of King Nut brand peanut butter.

On January 16, the Connecticut Department of Public Health Laboratory isolated the outbreak strain of *S*. Typhimurium from a previously unopened 5-pound container of King Nut creamy peanut butter, suggesting that contamination occurred during production. However, CDC's ongoing collaboration with states indicated that many cases did not eat peanut butter in institutions, but had eaten various other peanut butter-containing products. FDA investigators reported that the PCA facility in Blakely produced peanut butter and also peanut paste (made from ground roasted peanuts) and other peanut products, which were sold to many food companies for use as an ingredient in peanut butter-containing foods.

To better determine the association of illness with other peanut-butter containing foods, a second study was conducted by CDC and state and local health departments January 17-19 to further assess exposures in persons who did not live in institutions and had become ill since December 1. Preliminary analysis found that ill persons were more likely than non-ill persons to have eaten specific brands of prepackaged peanut butter crackers. Both brands of peanut butter crackers are made at one plant, which is known to receive peanut paste from PCA.

Intact packages of peanut butter crackers that had been purchased in the United States were obtained from the home of a patient in Canada by the Canadian Food Inspection Agency. Culture of a composite sample of the crackers yielded the outbreak strain of *S*. Typhimurium. Other testing of three intact packages of peanut butter crackers obtained from a patient's home in Oregon showed similar *Salmonella* contamination.

Throughout the investigative process, to ensure that information was disseminated to the public as accurately and quickly as possible about health threats and other information related to this outbreak, CDC and FDA coordinated their communication strategies and messages and discussed these strategies in daily calls with state health officials. We balance the rapid release of information on sources of illness against the potential negative consequences to consumers, food growers, producers, and industry. Continued collaborations and communications between federal agencies, state and local health departments, and all relevant stakeholders are essential.

Status of Investigation

As of February 1, 2009, 550 persons from 43 states and one person from Canada had been reported infected with the outbreak strain. Confirmed, reported onset of illness dates have ranged from September 1, 2008, to January 17, 2009. A total of 120 patients were reported hospitalized, and the infection may have contributed to eight deaths. The epidemiologic, laboratory, and traceback findings from this continuing investigation indicate that peanut butter and peanut paste produced at the PCA plant are the source of the outbreak. More specifically, the outbreak was caused by contaminated peanut butter used in institutions, and by peanut butter and peanut paste used as ingredients in food products. The second case-control study indicated a particular risk with peanut butter crackers, but this does not exonerate other peanut-containing products.

After one brand of peanut butter served in institutions was implicated by epidemiologic and laboratory evidence, the investigation was expanded to include food items that use peanut butter and peanut paste made in the same factory as ingredients in peanut butter-containing products. This was an ingredient-driven outbreak, in which a contaminated ingredient affected many different products that are distributed through various channels and consumed in various settings. Peanut butter and peanut paste are common ingredients in cookies, crackers, cereal, candy, ice cream, pet treats, and other foods. Mass food distribution can lead to widely distributed nationwide outbreaks.

CONCLUSION

The large number of products and brands recalled already, and the large quantities of some products recalled, makes this one of the largest recalls in the United States. The outbreak appears to be slowing, but we are not able to say that the outbreak is over at this point. Because of the time lag in reporting, we expect reports of new cases to continue for 2-3 weeks after the outbreak actually ends. The event illustrates how a large and widespread outbreak can occur, from distribution of a single item to hundreds of foods. It also highlights the continued need for robust disease detection systems at all levels—local, state, and federal—to ensure prompt recognition, response, and investigation of these outbreaks. CDC will continue its efforts to:

- focus on research, education, and training that will assist with Federal strategies to prevent foodborne illnesses before they happen;
- incorporate food industries into prevention, response and information sharing; and
- bolster state health infrastructures to effectively and promptly identify and respond to outbreaks.

This will entail continuing to work with regulatory authorities, state and local partners, food and environmental microbiologist scientists, and the food industry to prevent future food borne illness outbreaks. Thank you again for the invitation to testify before you today. I will be happy to answer any questions you may have.

In: The Salmonella Outbreak in Peanut Products: The FDA … ISBN: 978-1-60741-950-1
Editor: Benjamin K. Glynn

Chapter 14

OVERSIGHT IN PEANUT RECALL HEARING-MEUNIER (MOTHER) TESTIMONY

Gabrielle Meunier

Thank you Senator Leahy and Chairman Harkin, and the rest of the Committee for the opportunity to appear before you today and share the story of my son Christopher and our experience with the recent *Salmonella* outbreak and the peanut recall that followed.

On Thanksgiving night, November 25, 2008, my perfectly healthy and robust seven-year-old son, Christopher, spiked a very high fever, started throwing up, and having diarrhea. His father and I suspected it was the flu, as did our Pediatrician, so we limited his food and made sure he got plenty of fluids. Two days later Christopher's health deteriorated dramatically, he was severely ill and in tremendous pain; a pain that no child should ever have to experience and as a mother one that I will never forget as I sat by his bedside. We immediately called our Pediatrician who instructed us to bring him to the hospital.

We asked ourselves how in the world could a seemingly perfectly healthy child get so sick in such a short period? However, once the lab results finally came back and he was diagnosed with *Salmonella,* the picture became clearer. Thankfully, after days of antibiotics, anti-fungus drugs, and no food or drink, his wrecked body finally stabilized to a point where he could come home. This, after six days and nights filled with fear and unanswered questions.

Senators I could spend all day telling you about Christopher's terrible experience and the questions that still linger about the long-term ramifications for his health, but I would rather use my limited time here today to help make change and progress for the future. Some excellent ideas have already been proposed for improving our food safety system and I would like to add a few of my own, while highlighting some of the mistakes I witnessed firsthand during Christopher's ordeal. I must start by praising the first line of defenders in the fight against foodborne illness. Senators it is my experience that this is the only part of the foodborne illness safety system that works well.

TECHNOLOGY AND INFORMATION

First, and foremost I believe that technology is the key to making our foodborne illness response work better and in a cohesive manner. I believe there needs to be a national online foodborne illness database/registry that can be used by victims as soon as a *Salmonella* or other foodborne illness has been diagnosed. Such a tool would allow patients or their caregivers to log on to the registry and fill out a questionnaire about food eaten in the seven days prior to illness onset. This can be done while the patient is still in the hospital or in the Doctor's office. By doing this step immediately, the information is still fresh in the victim's mind rather than on the phone for a two and a half hour interview over a week after the initial diagnosis.

In this age of technology, text messages, and instant messaging; I do not understand why victims could not be given access to a secure website and chat-room to allow them to talk to one another and possibly solve the question of which food poisoned them. In Christopher's case, he is a very picky eater. I am chagrinned to say that my son mostly eats cheese, milk, yogurt, peanut butter, and snacks like chips, peanuts or crackers. Had I had an opportunity to talk to other mothers whose children were sick, and compare what they had eaten I have no doubt we could have cracked this case back in early December.

In addition to using technology to get information from victims, I feel that it can be used better for sharing information with victims and the public. In my opinion, the agencies involved with any outbreak should never underestimate how much victims and the public crave information. I was kept in the dark for way too long throughout this process, at one point having to insist that I be told what specific kind of *Salmonella* Christopher had, even though the health worker I was speaking to said that "I didn't need to know." The victims must be kept in the loop with real time information and there needs to be a way to reach all the victims by phone. I believe that a computerized phone message to victims could easily be established for disseminating information -- after all how many people in this room got text messages from the president during the inauguration weekend?

In this case, as soon as there was the slightest possibility that crackers and other foods were the culprit, we should have received a message telling us to remove any peanut butter crackers from our house. Thankfully, a coworker of mine read that tainted Crackers possibly contained Salmonella. Then it all made sense, Christopher had eaten a package of cheese and peanut butter crackers but no one else in our family had. This is where our case hit another roadblock, when I called the CDC about the crackers, which we still had in our pantry, no one would take my call. Thankfully, when I called the FDA, I found someone willing to listen, unfortunately it was the weekend and that Monday was a holiday so no one could pick up the crackers until Tuesday. However, in a shocking twist the woman I spoke with at the FDA then also wanted to give me a questionnaire about all the foods Christopher had eaten, all the same information I had already given the CDC. I do not understand why the various agencies working on this outbreak did not already have our information. Technology must be used to share information between all the teams and lines of defense working on an outbreak.

In addition to notifying victims, the public needs to be kept informed as well, perhaps with an alert system similar to those for storm warnings. This system could also be utilized to update the public when it is safe to eat a certain food again. Right now it has is a guessing game for the public – and sometimes just a game of Russian roulette.

Identification

Next, I believe there should be a unified procedure for the identification of all Salmonella cases. If one state does this best, then they should share their procedures and best practices with the rest of the country for the fastest turn around possible. Once identification is made and the data entered into the registry, the correlations can be made to determine if there is a pattern developing. If there is, then there is already a litany of information regarding foods eaten, already provided by the victims so swift action can be taken.

National Team

After our experience, I believe that there should be one team involved at the National level in charge of the follow up. Such a national team could again use technology and the registry/database for all their information dissemination to all lines of defense and data gathering. It is crucial that four lines of defense have access to the information on the database, this includes the local Doctors and hospitals, the State Health Departments, the CDC, and finally the FDA. With one team involved in tracking and organizing the investigation, if any sort of clusters or patterns are identified by that team, this information can be shared to all parties through the registry database.

As the system is now, Christopher's doctors had to ask around on their own if other local pediatricians had patients with similar symptoms. Had there been a national database, they would have seen that on the date that Christopher was diagnosed, that there was already a cluster of Salmonella elsewhere in the U.S. They could have then seen if there were any other cases in Vermont. This information is important for the first lines of defense to have – even if does not effect their specific region of care. If we were to have a Bioterrorist act through food, this data would be invaluable information to all lines of defense.

Personal Responsibility

Finally, I believe there needs to be personal responsibility in manufacturing and growing foods for consumption by the public. The owners of companies must be personally responsible for the safety of the foods they sell. Inspection records should online and made available to the general public, owners should have to log-on to a database at regular intervals, depending on the amount of products produced, and personally attest to the safety of their food.

Manufacturers must take responsibility for all items that go into their products, and therefore if they are purchasing supplies and ingredients from other companies, they need to attest and be equally responsible for that ingredient as well. If their supplier is listed on a public database and personally attesting for the safety of their product then their liability for that supplier is lowered if their supplier is meeting all required standards. In this particular case, there has rightfully been a lot of blame placed on the plant where the contaminated product originated, however I believe that large suppliers of food products, should have a clear process to verify that their suppliers are meeting national standards. Clearly, that did not happen in this case, and now the government must ensure this will never happen again.

Thank you again to the committee for holding this hearing today. I would like to close by thanking the Staff at the Children's Hospital of Vermont for treating Christopher so promptly. Our family is so thankful that he received the best care in the world and lucky for us he was a big boy to begin with. I shudder to think of the outcome had he been an underweight or sickly child to begin with and my heart goes out to all of the other victims and their families.

Again, thank you and I welcome any questions you may have.

In: The Salmonella Outbreak in Peanut Products: The FDA … ISBN: 978-1-60741-950-1
Editor: Benjamin K. Glynn

Chapter 15

Oversight in Peanut Recall Hearing-Sundlof (FDA) Testimony

Stephen F. Sundlof

Introduction

Good morning Mr. Chairman and members of the Committee. I am Dr. Stephen Sundlof, Director of the Center for Food Safety and Applied Nutrition at the U.S. Food and Drug Administration (FDA or the Agency), which is part of the Department of Health and Human Services. FDA appreciates the opportunity to provide you with information on our ongoing investigation of the foodborne illness outbreak associated with *Salmonella* Typhimurium, which has been found in peanut products produced by the Peanut Corporation of America (PCA). Because our investigation and the accompanying recall of suspect product continues as we speak, our final conclusions and recommendations are necessarily pending the outcome of our investigation.

Let me begin by providing a brief description of the typical traceback process employed by FDA and our sister agency, the Centers for Disease Control and Prevention (CDC). Once CDC, through its epidemiological investigation which involves working with state and local health departments, identifies the possible food(s) associated with a foodborne illness outbreak, CDC notifies FDA. At that point, FDA considers the strength of the evidence implicating the suspect food or foods and determines the appropriate level of regulatory response. To start our traceback investigation to identify the source of the contamination, we work with the food industry and with state and local regulatory partners, and, when needed, with foreign governments. We do this by tracing the food suspected of being the vehicle for transmitting the pathogen back through the supply chain from the retailer, restaurant or institutional setting and inspecting or investigating points throughout the supply chain to determine where the contamination most likely occurred. Tracing food requires us to find and examine documentation (such as bills of lading and invoices) for the product throughout the supply chain. We also obtain information on the practices and conditions under which the product was stored and handled at each point to better determine shipments of interest and whether contamination may have occurred at each point. The records we need are not always in an electronic format, and records review often can be a time-consuming, resource intensive process.

In the current case, FDA began its investigation prior to having a strong epidemiological link to a particular food, both to inform the epidemiological study and to shorten the time required to get potentially contaminated foods off the market. Because institutionally-served peanut butter, in five-pound containers, was identified by the state of Minnesota as a potential vehicle, our investigation had a strong lead: the brand name of a company and the address to begin our trace. But allow me to explain a few components of the epidemiological work, the first step in our collaborative efforts.

Epidemiological Investigation

Since early December 2008, FDA has collaborated with CDC, the Food Safety and Inspection Service (FSIS) of the United States Department of Agriculture (USDA), and public health officials in various states to investigate the multi-state outbreak of human infections due to *Salmonella* Typhimurium. Early epidemiological efforts to identify a likely food vehicle were inconclusive. While initial efforts focused on the potential for chicken to be the illness vehicle, peanut butter was first identified as a possible source in mid-December. On January 7 and 8, after conversations with CDC, FSIS, and the Minnesota Department of Health about the strength of association between illness and exposure to chicken or peanut butter, FDA decided to begin to investigate institutional food service sources of peanut butter despite the inconclusive epidemiological data.

On January 7, based on preliminary information from CDC's multi-state case control study that explored other possible food sources in addition to peanut butter, and before Minnesota had identified the *Salmonella* strain, FDA made its initial contact with the King Nut Company in Ohio. King Nut distributes peanut butter manufactured by the Peanut Corporation of America (PCA) at its Blakely, Georgia, plant to institutional facilities, food service industries, and private label food companies in several states. On January 9, FDA initiated an inspection of the PCA plant in Blakely, and Minnesota reported that they had isolated *Salmonella* from the open container, though the type of *Salmonella* was not yet known.

As part of its epidemiological investigation, the Minnesota Department of Health tested an open five-pound container of King Nut peanut butter obtained at a nursing home where three patients were sickened by the outbreak strain of *Salmonella* Typhimurium. By January 10, Minnesota health officials had determined that the peanut butter contained the same strain of *Salmonella* Typhimurium associated with the illnesses linked to the outbreak. However, because it is always possible that the open container was contaminated by someone or something else in the environment, these results did not definitively confirm PCA as the source. FDA and other state health departments expanded the testing of unopened containers of the same brand of peanut butter.

On January 19, testing by the Connecticut Department of Health of an unopened container of King Nut peanut butter showed that it contained the same strain of *Salmonella* Typhimurium associated with illnesses linked to the outbreak. The fact that the *Salmonella*

Typhimurium was confirmed in an unopened container of peanut butter indicated that the peanut butter was contaminated when it left the Blakely processing plant.

Peanut butter is sold by PCA in bulk containers ranging in size from five to 1,700 pounds. The peanut paste is sold in sizes ranging from 35-pound containers to tanker trucks. However, through its investigation, FDA has determined that PCA distributed potentially contaminated products to more than 300 consignee firms, many of whom then further distributed products, for consumption as peanut butter or for use as ingredients in hundreds of different products, such as cookies, crackers, cereal, candy and ice cream.

As of February 1, CDC reported that 550 persons infected with the outbreak strain of *Salmonella* Typhimurium have been reported from 43 states, plus one person from Canada, and that the infection may have contributed to eight deaths.

Plant Inspection

After visiting King Nut on January 8 to determine where its peanut butter was manufactured and to collect samples, FDA initiated an inspection of PCA's Blakely plant on January 9, shortly after preliminary information indicated that this firm might be linked to the ongoing *Salmonella* outbreak. FDA completed its inspection on January 27.

A document listing observations by FDA investigators during their inspection, known as a List of Inspectional Observations, or Form 483, has been posted on FDA's website at www.fda.gov/ora/frequent/default.htm. This list is not a final Agency determination regarding compliance. The list of observations includes matters relating to cleaning programs and procedures as well as failure to implement steps to mitigate *Salmonella* contamination in the facility.

FDA's environmental sampling at the plant found two *Salmonella* strains, neither of which were *Salmonella* Typhimurium, the outbreak strain. As of now, CDC is not aware of any illnesses definitely connected to these other *Salmonella* strains. We are confident, however, based on the investigations by the states, CDC and FDA, including product testing, that the Blakely plant is the source of the contaminated foods related to the current *Salmonella* Typhimurium outbreak. State sampling and analysis of unopened finished products indicate that PCA-shipped product from the Blakely plant was contaminated with the outbreak strain.

Further, FDA's review of the firm's testing records -- which were not disclosed to FDA and state inspectors during earlier routine inspections -- revealed that there were instances in 2007 and 2008 where the firm distributed product in commerce which tested positive for *Salmonella*.

As you may be aware, FDA has recently confirmed that our Office of Criminal Investigations (OCI) is conducting an ongoing criminal investigation.

Product Recalls

After discussions with FDA, the first product recall related to the outbreak was initiated on January 10, 2009, by the King Nut Company of peanut butter distributed under the King

Nut and Parnell's Pride labels. On January 13, PCA initiated a voluntary recall of certain lots of peanut butter and peanut paste produced on or after July 1, 2008, due to the risk of *Salmonella* contamination. PCA expanded this recall on January 16 to include peanut butter produced on or after August 8, 2009, and peanut paste produced on or after September 26, 2008. This was followed by yet another expansion on January 18, 2008, when PCA announced it was recalling all peanut butter and peanut paste manufactured on or after July 1, 2008, at its Blakely processing plant.

On January 28, PCA issued another expanded voluntary recall of all peanuts and peanut products, including all peanuts (dry and oil roasted), granulated peanuts, peanut meal, peanut butter and peanut paste processed in its Blakely facility since January 1, 2007. All of these recalled peanuts and peanut products were made only at the company's Blakely facility.

Many companies that received peanuts and peanut products manufactured by PCA's Blakely facility have, in turn, conducted voluntary recalls. A user-friendly, searchable list of the products being recalled, with corresponding photographs, when available, can be found at www.accessdata.fda.gov/scripts. The searchable list currently includes approximately 1,000 entries in 16 categories representing products that have been recalled by more than 75 companies. FDA is updating this list on a daily basis, as new information becomes available.

FDA has been working with purchasers of PCA's peanuts and peanut products to identify affected products and facilitate their removal from the market. FDA initiated inspections at the direct consignees of PCA and King Nut and continues to follow the distribution points for products. FDA and state officials have contacted hundreds of firms throughout the entire distribution chain that may have purchased or further distributed PCA products. This work is continuing and includes the additional products in the expanded recall.

Companies nationwide that received product made by PCA have issued voluntary recalls of their products. As FDA gathers additional information about these products, the list of recalled products has expanded, and will likely continue to do so. FDA urges all affected retailers to immediately stop selling recalled products. Directors of institutions and food service establishments are also strongly urged to ensure that they are not serving recalled products.

We would like to emphasize, as we have stated numerous times, that major national brands of jarred peanut butter found in grocery stores are not affected by the PCA recall. Further, FDA has no evidence to suggest that the *Salmonella* Typhimurium contamination originated with any manufacturing facility other than PCA's Blakely plant. The facility is not operating at this time.

Recommendations for Consumers

FDA has established a web page to provide constantly updated information on the contamination and recall at www.fda.gov/oc/opacom/hottopics/salmonellatyph.html. This web page has already been viewed more than 19 million times. The web page includes a searchable database to assist consumers in quickly identifying recalled products, found at www.accessdata.fda.gov/scripts

Consumers are urged to check this web page to determine which products have been recalled and to become aware of new recalls as they are announced. Any product that is on the recall list should be disposed of in a safe manner. Consumers are also urged to wash their hands after handling potentially contaminated products. If consumers are unsure whether a peanut- containing product is potentially contaminated, they should avoid consuming it until they obtain more information about the product. Persons who think they may have become ill from eating peanut products are advised to consult their health care providers.

Product recalls include some pet food products that contain peanut products made by PCA. Although the risk of animals contracting salmonellosis is minimal, there is risk to humans from handling these products. It is important for people to wash their hands -- and make sure children wash their hands -- before and, especially, after feeding pets. Further information for consumers is located in the Frequently Asked Questions section located on this web site. The pet food products are also included in the searchable data base of recalled products.

For information on products containing peanut butter from companies not reporting recalls, consumers may wish to consult the company's website or call the toll-free number listed on most packaging. We note that information consumers may receive from the companies has not been verified by FDA.

Product Manufacturers and Distributors

FDA urges manufacturers and distributors of products containing peanut-based ingredients to inform consumers about whether their products could contain peanuts or peanut products from PCA Blakely. If a manufacturer knows its products do not contain peanuts or peanut products from PCA, it may wish to provide this information to consumers.

FDA is continuing to work with the firms on the details of their actions, conducting follow-up audits and inspections, monitoring the progress of the firms' actions, working with state and local regulatory authorities, and notifying our foreign regulatory counterparts of products that have now been confirmed as having been distributed internationally. FDA is continuing its work to identify products that may be affected, and to track the ingredient supply chain of those products to facilitate their removal from the marketplace.

Conclusion

FDA is working hard to ensure the safety of food, in collaboration with its Federal, state, local, and international food safety partners, and with industry, consumers, and academia. Although the *Salmonella* Typhimurium foodborne illness outbreak underscores the challenges we face, the American food supply continues to be among the safest in the world. Food safety is a priority for the new Administration.

Over the last year and a half, FDA has made significant progress in identifying food vulnerabilities and mitigation strategies. For example, we have strengthened our response to food safety threats by providing incident command system training to our FDA offices around the country, and to states, and by developing templates to enhance communication during a food recall. We are proud of the collaborative efforts among Federal and state agencies to investigate, analyze samples, monitor the effectiveness of the current recall, and communicate with the public to protect public health. We will continue to strive to reduce the incidence of foodborne illness to the lowest level possible.

Thank you for the opportunity to discuss FDA's response to the recent *Salmonella* outbreak. I would be happy to answer any questions you may have.

In: The Salmonella Outbreak in Peanut Products: The FDA … ISBN: 978-1-60741-950-1
Editor: Benjamin K. Glynn

Chapter 16

SALMONELLA & INDUSTRY ROLE IN PROTECTION HEARING- WAXMAN STATEMENT

Henry A. Waxman

Thank you, Chairman Stupak. I want to commend you for your hard work on this investigation and for keeping the focus squarely where it belongs: on the glaring holes at all levels of our food safety network.

Today is the third hearing on these issues before the Energy and Commerce Committee. At our first hearing on February 11, it was clear that the Peanut Corporation of America was more interested in its financial well-being than the health and safety of its customers.

Rather than expressions of regret or sorrow for the illnesses the company caused, we saw internal communications complaining about the impact that positive *salmonella* tests were having on the company's bottom line.

We also received testimony from FDA about basic authorities it currently lacks. FDA does not have the authority to routinely access records documenting the steps manufacturers take to assure safety. FDA cannot order a company to recall dangerous food products — it can only make a request and hope the company complies.

On March 11, we held our Committee's second hearing, before the Subcommittee on Health. At that hearing, witnesses explained that FDA cannot solve these critical problems alone. There are over 300,000 registered food facilities throughout the U.S. and abroad, and we cannot expect FDA to prevent food borne illness through inspections or post hoc investigations.

Today we will examine the role of industry in protecting our nation's food supply. We will hear from three companies that purchased peanut products from PCA, despite the filthy conditions at its plants in Georgia and Texas.

These companies used PCA ingredients that were tainted with *salmonella.* They included them in their own products under their own labels, and they caused illnesses and in some cases even death, according to state and federal officials.

At our February hearing, Dr. Stephen Sundlof, FDA's Director of Food Safety and Applied Nutrition, agreed that "each company in the chain of manufacturing has an obligation to ensure that the ingredients they are using as well as their final products are safe for Americans to consume."

I wholeheartedly agree. But, as we will see today, all three companies failed to meet this standard. Their final products were not safe, and people suffered as a result.

Let me make one final point. Some of today's witnesses, and many companies like them, relied on third party auditors to inspect the facilities of their suppliers. This hearing will expose some of the dangers related to this system. I raised serious concerns about this at our hearing last week.

If we are going to consider a third party system, we must, at minimum, ensure it addresses the serious problems we will hear about today. But there are additional problems this hearing won't address, such as using foreign third parties to inspect foods we import from other countries. This Committee will be looking closely at all of these issues in the coming weeks.

In this case, a private, for-profit auditing firm called AIB gave PCA glowing reviews. This company was selected by PCA, it was paid by PCA, and it reported to PCA.

Let me show you an award it gave to PCA on August 20, 2008. This "certificate of achievement" was given to PCA's Texas plant for fulfilling "the requirements of the AIB Consolidated Standards for Food Safety."

And you can see the "superior" rating between the signatures of AIB's President and the Chairman of the Board.

We've all now seen the pictures of what this Texas plant was really like: rodents, excrement, and filth.

How could a facility that was in such deplorable conditions receive such glowing reviews?

And how is it possible that any of our witnesses could have relied on such flawed inspections?

We will have hard questions for our witnesses today, but we also thank them for their cooperation. They provided thousands of pages of documents to the Committee, and they helped state and federal authorities remove deadly products from family kitchens across the country.

Our goal now is to develop common sense legislation to improve preventive systems at the front end of this process before one more person dies from tainted food.

In: The Salmonella Outbreak in Peanut Products: The FDA … ISBN: 978-1-60741-950-1
Editor: Benjamin K. Glynn

Chapter 17

SALMONELLA & INDUSTRY ROLE IN PROTECTION HEARING- STUPAK STATEMENT

Bart Stupak

"Mold was observed growing on the ceiling and walls"... "rain water was observed dripping into the plant's peanut processing areas"... "6 dead mice were found in the false ceiling area"... air filters were "littered with feathers"... "a live roach and several dead roaches were observed in the firm's wash room"... "REPs [rodent excreta pellets] too numerous to count were observed."

The pictures you are seeing, and the quotes I am reading, come from federal inspections of facilities in Georgia and Texas operated by the Peanut Corporation of America. At the Subcommittee's first hearing on February 11, 2009, we heard testimony about filthy conditions and at least a dozen positive salmonella tests that PCA received in 2007 and 2008.

Today, the Subcommittee will continue its investigation by hearing from representatives of three companies that bought products from these polluted PCA facilities: the Kellogg Company, the King Nut Company, and Vitamin Cottage Natural Food Markets.

We will ask a series of questions today. First, we will ask why their food safety procedures failed to prevent the contamination of their products.

The written testimony submitted for today's hearing suggests that some of the companies believe PCA was entirely at fault, and that they should not be held responsible for the safety of ingredients they bought from a disreputable supplier. PCA certainly deserves its share of the blame, and there are ongoing criminal investigations of its actions.

But all three of these companies put their own labels on these products. They put their names on them. They represented to the public that these products were safe to eat. And they sold them to consumers who became ill and in some cases died, according to state and federal authorities.

Placing all the blame on PCA would mean that food processors have no responsibility for ensuring the safety of their ingredients. And I simply can't agree with that.

Second, we will ask whether these companies should have known or suspected problems with PCA before the outbreak. In written testimony submitted today, Martin Kanan, the

President and CEO of King Nut, states that PCA's president, Stewart Parnell, informed King Nut on January 7, 2009, that he had no knowledge of any salmonella issues with his products.

The documents tell a different story. On the same day, January 7, Mr. Parnell sent an e-mail to King Nut's Vice President for Finance and Administration, Joe Valenza.

In this e-mail, PCA's president, Mr. Parnell, forwarded a news account of the emerging outbreak to King Nut's Vice President and said, "Joe, I'm sure it's something we did." Eleven minutes later, King Nut's Vice President replied: "I'm recalling everything." Four minutes later, Mr. Parnell replied: "Now my heart is really in my throat. I think I'm going to church tonight."

Third, we will ask why none of these companies ever asked PCA officials to disclose their positive tests for salmonella. If your supplier tests positive, this is definitely something you should find out, and it's certainly something your customers deserve to know.

Even industry insiders recognized this. In an e-mail on February 5, 2009, an official at a private food safety auditing firm wrote to a co-worker: "[T]he biggest problem was with the positive micro data that they ignored. ... this data was not initially available for the FDA either. They had to really pry into their documentation before uncovering the additional test results."

Fourth, we will ask why these companies relied on audits by AIB, a firm that was selected and paid by PCA. There is an obvious and inherent conflict of interest when an auditor works for the same supplier it is evaluating, and several documents show evidence of this cozy relationship.

On December 22, 2008, PCA's auditor e-mailed Sammy Lightsey, the manager of PCA's Georgia plant, to give him advance notice of an upcoming inspection. He stated: "You lucky guy. I am your AIB auditor. So we need to get your plant set up for any audit." The result of that audit was a rating of "superior."

The conclusions were completely different when the auditors were not paid by PCA. Today, we will release several audits that have not yet been made public. They were conducted not by the auditor PCA hired, but by internal auditors working for Nestle USA.

In 2002, Nestle auditors found that PCA's Georgia facility had no plan to address microbiological hazards like salmonella. Their audit found a "potential for microbiological cross contamination" and concluded that PCA was "not in compliance" with housekeeping, sanitation, and pest control standards. The audit noted:

"Rodent droppings in the break room cabinets"
"Live Flour beetle activity in the blancher room"
"Dead Flour beetles found in stored screens in the bleacher room"
"Dead insects found on the interior perimeters"

The audit warned that "it is critical that these deficiencies are addressed." But its findings in 2002 were similar to those of federal investigators seven years later.

Nestle USA also conducted an audit of PCA's Texas facility in 2006 and came to similar conclusions. As a result, Nestle USA rejected PCA as a supplier. We will ask the other companies here today why they did not do the same. If they had, perhaps some of these illnesses and deaths would have been avoided.

In conclusion, I ask unanimous consent that the documents in my opening statement and in the binder prepared by staff be entered into the official hearing record.

In: The Salmonella Outbreak in Peanut Products: The FDA … ISBN: 978-1-60741-950-1
Editor: Benjamin K. Glynn

Chapter 18

SALMONELLA & INDUSTRY ROLE IN PROTECTION HEARING- STUPAK IMAGES

Benjamin K. Glynn

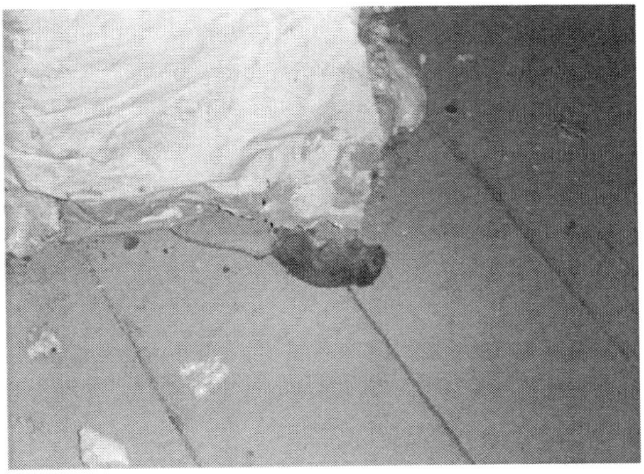

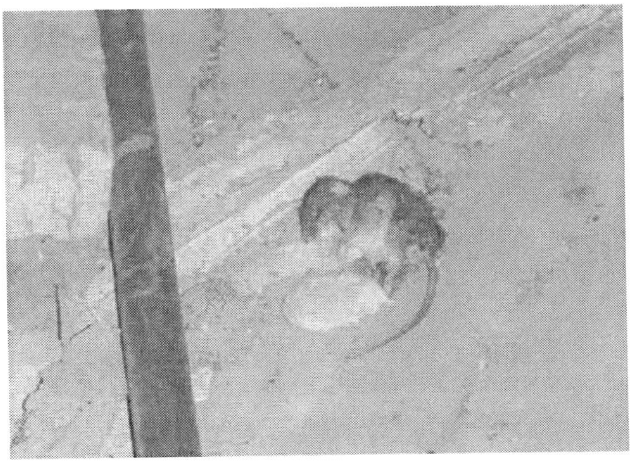

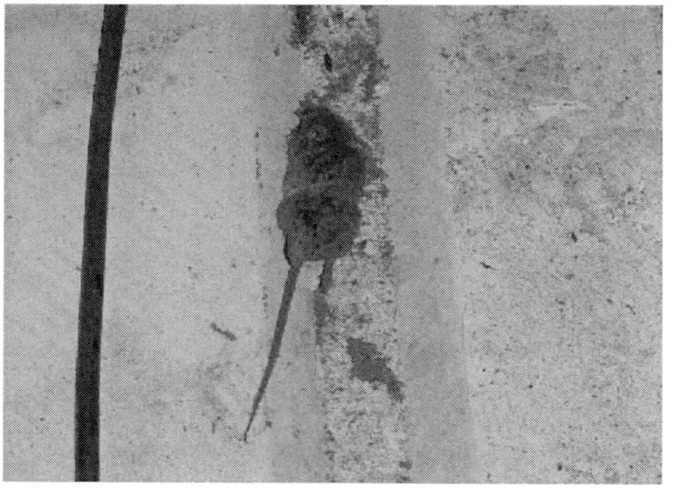

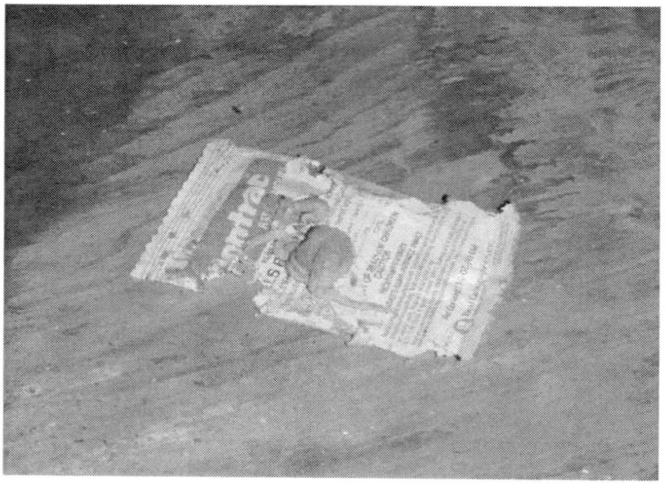

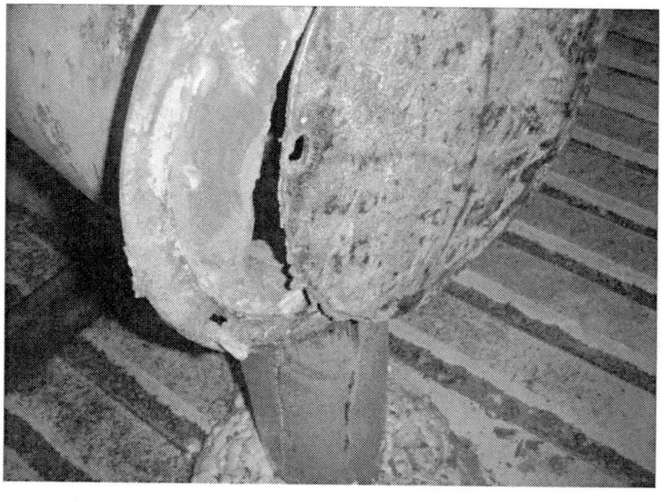

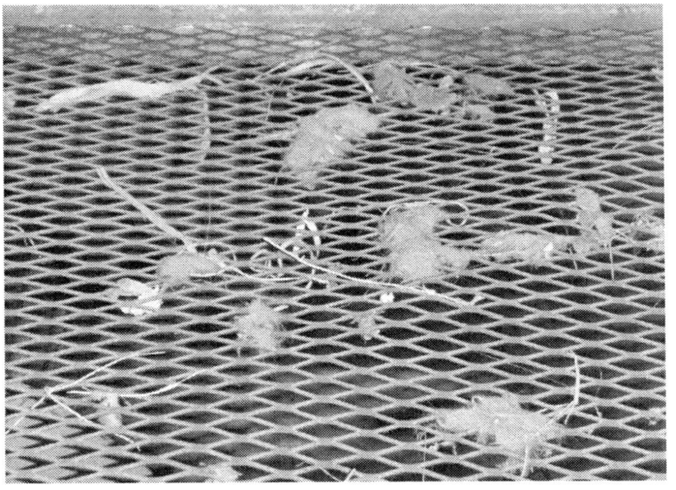

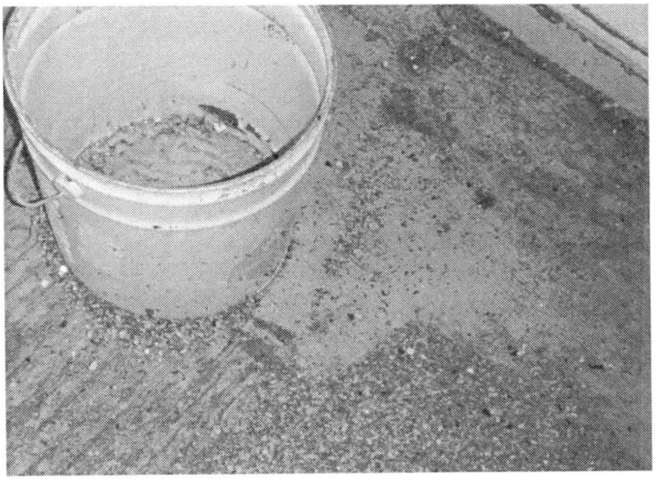

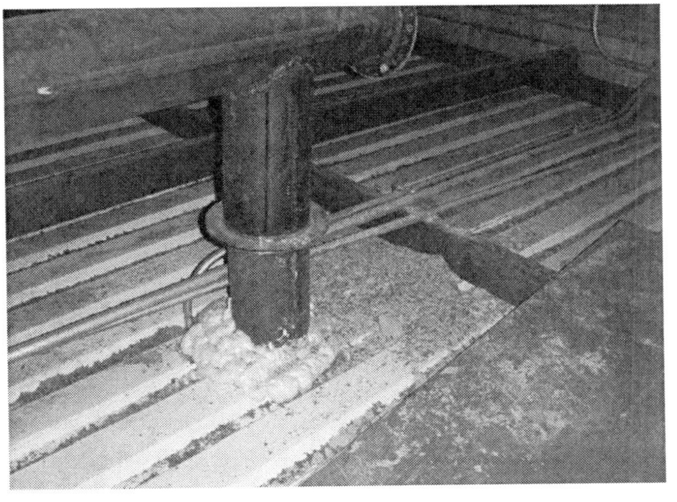

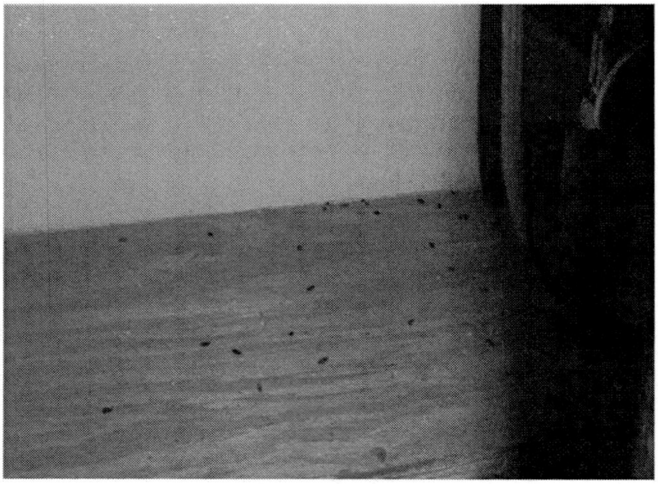

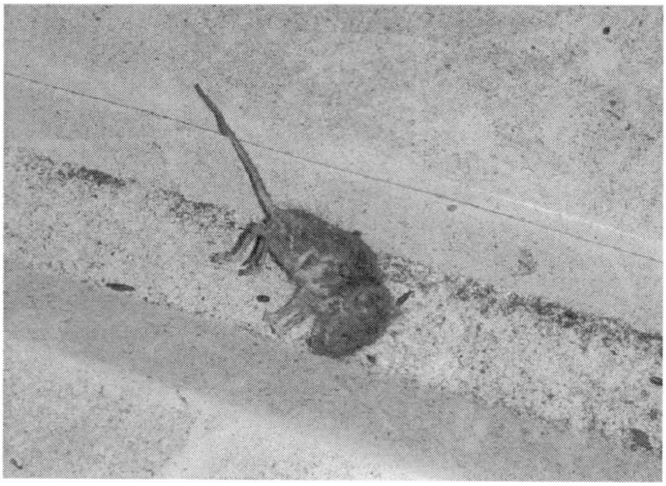

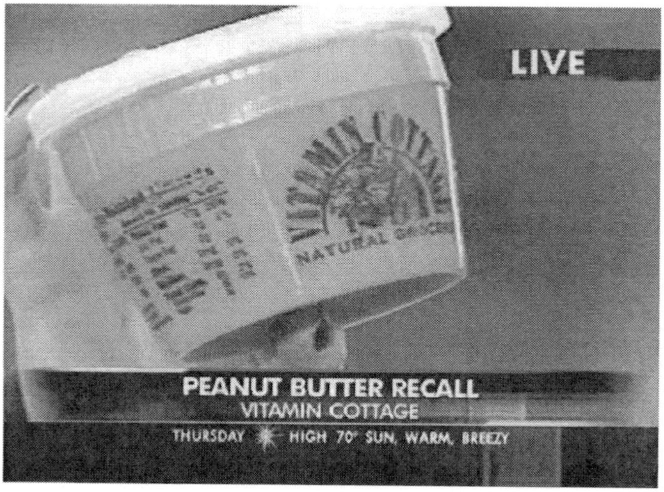
LIVE
PEANUT BUTTER RECALL
VITAMIN COTTAGE
THURSDAY HIGH 70° SUN, WARM, BREEZY

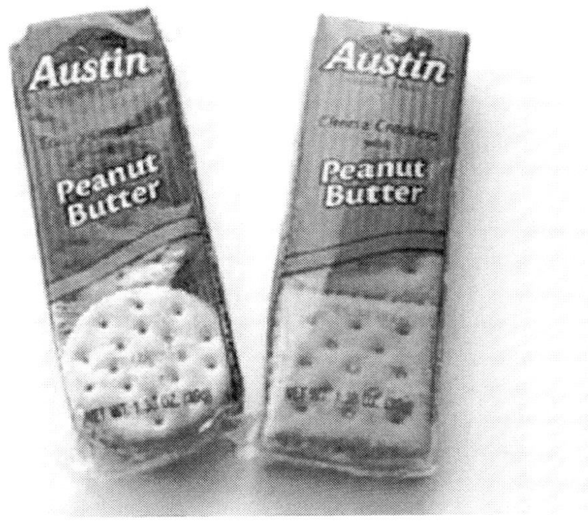

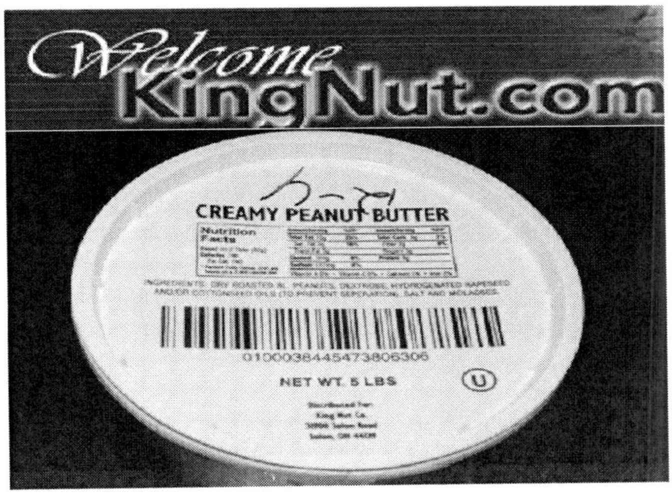

Parnell: "Joe, I'm sure it's something we did."
Valenza: "I'm recalling everything."
Parnell: "Now my heart is really in my throat. I think I'm going to church tonight."

Stewart Parnell and Joe Valenza,
January 7, 2009

"[T]he biggest problem was with the positive micro data that they ignored. ... this data was not initially available for the FDA either. They had to really pry into their documentation before uncovering the additional test results."

NSF Official, February 5, 2009

"You lucky guy. I am your AIB auditor. So we need to get your plant set up for any audit."

Pete Hatfield to Sammy
Lightsey, December 22, 2008

Rodent droppings in the break room cabinets
Live Flour beetle activity in the blancher room
Dead Flour beetles found in stored screens in the bleacher room
Dead insects found on the interior perimeters

Nestle USA Audit, 2002

In: The Salmonella Outbreak in Peanut Products: The FDA … ISBN: 978-1-60741-950-1
Editor: Benjamin K. Glynn

Chapter 19

SALMONELLA & INDUSTRY ROLE IN PROTECTION HEARING-KANAN TESTIMONY

J. Martin Kanan

INTRODUCTION

Good morning Mr. Chairman and members of the Subcommittee. My name is Martin Kanan and I am President and CEO of Kanan Enterprises, Inc. Since 1989, Kanan Enterprises, my family owned business, has done business as King Nut Company. We are proud that the operating companies that my family now owns started in 1927 and 1937 in Cleveland, Ohio. We are a leading national supplier of snack nuts and other items to airline, retail, vending, food service, gift and private label industries.

I understand that today's hearing is to investigate the safety of the nation's food supply and specifically to examine the recent *Salmonella* outbreak associated with peanut products manufactured by the Peanut Corporation of America (PCA). Let me begin by stating something that you've heard many times before from others in the food industry, and will hopefully hear many times in the future: The health and safety of those who consume our products is our first priority. Food safety is paramount.

That is why Kanan Enterprises has always and will always regularly review and analyze its processes, procedures, plans and actions to identify lessons learned and areas for improvement. Such continuous improvement is how Kanan Enterprises grew from 25 employees in 1989 to almost 200 today. Our union run facilities, by the proud Teamsters Union, produce nearly 500 million bags of product per year. None of which is associated with this outbreak. With the growth in volume of product, we also grew in our sophistication on other aspects of the business. However, we have never lost sight and we will never loose sight that the key to longevity is producing safe, wholesome, quality food items.

The recent Salmonella outbreak is a tragedy for all of the victims, their families and the food industry. Thus, I will share with this subcommittee our relationship with Peanut Corporation of America and our role in being the first to recall PCA's peanut butter.

Relationship With Peanut Corporation of America

As our business expanded, our foodservice customers began asking us if we would supply them with peanut butter. Our customers wanted industrial sized peanut butter, 5 lb and 35 lb containers. However, we are not a peanut butter manufacturer. To help us find a peanut butter manufacturer, we enlisted one of our long standing peanut brokers and asked that our broker find a peanut butter manufacturer that would "private label" the finished product for us. Private labeling for us meant that the manufacturer would sell us a high quality, finished, sealed product packaged with our label in a closed and finished case. Kanan would not manufacture, process or package the peanut butter.

Our first supplier of peanut butter had issues meeting a good consistency in the product, so our customers asked us to change. In early 2004, our peanut broker then presented PCA to us. In the peanut products industry, PCA is very well known and PCA had supplied, among others, a world leading food manufacturer. In 2004, PCA started as King Nut's private labeler. Over the years, PCA private labeled King Nut's 5 lb creamy and crunchy peanut butter. Kanan also purchased from PCA, Parnell's Pride which is a 35 lb creamy peanut butter.

Throughout the 5 years of doing business with PCA, we received PCA's specification sheets for the products. The specification required, among many other microbiological requirements, no Salmonella to be present in the product, which we understood would be confirmed by testing. We've learned that contamination of peanut butter with *Salmonella* is usually an issue of recontamination after the roasting process. Such contamination would normally be dealt with through the application of GMP measures including sanitation and separation of finished product from raw materials.

In addition to product specification sheets, we received several Continuing Pure Food Guarantees from PCA. These Guarantees affirmatively stated that PCA guaranteed that any product shipped by PCA to Kanan was produced in accordance with good manufacturing practices, was unadulterated, safe and free of any substance which was in any way injurious. These Continuing Pure Food Guarantees were backed up by certificates of insurance, a Total Quality Systems Audit Report Summary, a letter from Stewart Parnell, PCA's President, extolling a Superior Rating from A.I.B. (American Institute of Baking) and assurances that PCA had a HACCP food safety plan in place. Late in the relationship, we received Certificates of Analysis or COA's. These COA's showed negative results for *Salmonella.*

At the end of 2008, Kanan distributed the PCA-manufactured and packaged peanut butter to seven foodservice distributors. Kanan never opened or altered the sealed containers of peanut butter. We did not suspect any health, safety or quality issues existed with PCA product until we were contacted on January 7, 2009, by the Minnesota Department of Agriculture.

Recall

We were the first in the United States to do a voluntary recall for any product associated with the recent *Salmonella* outbreak. The timeline on the recall began with a call from the Minnesota Department of Agriculture. On Wednesday, January 7, 2009, they informed us that they were investigating *Salmonella* incidents and wanted to know who manufactured the King

Nut peanut butter. We told them that it was PCA. We contacted the broker for PCA and requested that PCA be informed of the investigation into the product. In response, Stewart Parnell, President of PCA, let us know that he had no knowledge of any *Salmonella* issue.

On Thursday, January 8, 2009, FDA investigators came to our facilities and stated they were in the early stages of investigation. We produced the bills of lading and the COA's from PCA for the peanut butter and they inventoried the lots of peanut butter we had in our warehouse. At that time we requested the FDA take samples of the peanut butter to test, but they declined to take test samples. Therefore, on that same day, we sent samples of the lots of peanut butter that we had in our warehouse to be tested for salmonella. On January 8, 2009, we also received a second call from the Minnesota Department of Agriculture informing us that peanut butter was a possible suspect and that samples from an open container had been sent for testing.

On Friday, January 9, 2009, the FDA investigators returned to our facility and we again answered questions regarding who manufactured the peanut butter. We informed them that we did not use peanut butter in any of the products we manufactured. Several hours later, the FDA investigators took samples of the peanut butter in our warehouse for testing.

At 4:30 pm on Friday, January 9, 2009, we received news from the Minnesota Department of Agriculture that the sampling from the open container of peanut butter had a presumptive positive for *Salmonella* and that the sub-type would not be confirmed until the following week. Even though it was a single open container and even though it was only a presumptive positive, my company took this very seriously. We wanted to protect the public. We did not want to wait for PCA to initiate a recall.

Prior to noon on Saturday, January 10, 2009, we initiated the first product recall related to the *Salmonella* outbreak. We recalled all of the PCA peanut butter that King Nut distributed in 2008, both King Nut and Parnell's Pride labels. Again, even though we were only a distributor, we did the recall without PCA as we believed it was the right thing to do. Our biggest concern was for the health and safety of the consumers of the products.

Under our recall system, we are able to communicate with our customers within approximately 45 minutes. All of our customers, the 7 foodservice distributors, were aware of the recall by the afternoon of January 10. On January 10, 2009, we also issued a nationwide press release as we did not know who might be the ultimate end consumer of the product.

On Monday, January 12, 2009, FDA investigators again came to gather more information about the recalled peanut butter and we provided them with all records they requested. We were also called and informed that 4 of the 13 samples from the open container of peanut butter in Minnesota had tested positive for *Salmonella* Typhimurium. This confirmed that our quick reaction to the presumptive positive was the right thing to do.

On January 13, 2009, PCA initiated a voluntary recall of certain lots of peanut butter and peanut paste produced on or after July 1, 2008, due to the risk of *Salmonella* contamination. As this SubCommittee is aware, PCA's recall has been expanded several times.

On January 29, 2009, we along with those in our industry and the consumers were shocked and dismayed at the findings that reported PCA knowingly released product with potential *Salmonella* contamination into the food supply.

The test results from our January 8 samples showed no *Salmonella* in the product. To this day, we have not been informed by the FDA or anyone else what the test results showed from the samples the FDA investigators took on January 9 from our warehouse.

RECOMMENDATIONS

The issue of food safety and the questions concerning the breakdowns in the food safety system have brought into question whether America's food supply is safe. This question is much broader than the recent *Salmonella* outbreak associated with PCA's peanut products. While I believe that the American food supply is one of the safest in the world, Kanan Enterprises continues to be committed to work to rebuild public confidence in the American food safety system, including both governmental oversight and manufacturing accountability. I want the food safety system to work and I want to be part of making things better for our country's food supply.

In the specific case of PCA, however, Kanan Enterprises must reiterate that it did not have control over the production or processing of the product, PCA did. PCA had guaranteed Kanan that its peanut butter would not have *Salmonella.* While most food manufacturers practice safe production, storage and handling of food ingredients, it is apparent that if someone lacks integrity and honesty they will be able to find ways to bypass any quality control or food safety system. I believe any system created by Congress will necessarily have to keep the public confidence by showing that even if something does go terribly wrong, the system reacts to correct it swiftly and punishes the wrong doer.

Food manufacturers bear the responsibility of safe food. As a responsible food manufacturer. I abide by the rules and expect all to abide by the rules.

CONCLUSION

This is a tragedy for all those involved - the victims, their families and our industry. Even though we would not have wanted to be thrown into this spotlight, I thank you for the opportunity to discuss these issues with you and would be happy to answer any question that you have.

In: The Salmonella Outbreak in Peanut Products: The FDA … ISBN: 978-1-60741-950-1
Editor: Benjamin K. Glynn

Chapter 20

Salmonella & Industry Role in Protection Hearing-Mackay Testimony

A. D. David Mackay

Introduction

Good Morning Mr. Chairman and members of the Subcommittee. I am David Mackay, President and CEO of the Kellogg Company. Kellogg is the world's leading producer of cereal and a leading producer of convenience foods, including cookies, crackers, toaster pastries, cereal bars, fruit snacks, frozen waffles and veggie foods. The company's brands include *Kellogg's®, Keebler®, Pop-Tarts®, Eggo®, Cheez-It®, Nutri-Grain®, Special K®, Bear Naked®, Kashi®, Rice Krispies®, Murray®, Austin®, Morningstar Farms®, Famous Amos®, Carr's®, Plantation®* and *Ready Crust®*. Our company began with 44 employees in Battle Creek, Michigan in 1906. Today we employ more than 32,000 people and sell our products in more than 180 countries around the world.

Kellogg has been bringing our best to consumers for more than 100 years. We have a longstanding commitment to upholding the highest quality in our operations. It is what our consumers and customers expect and what we strive to deliver.

First and foremost, we deeply regret that the recent Salmonella recall situation occurred and that it involved Kellogg's products. We apologize to our customers and consumers, especially to those who may have become ill from one of our products.

We, just like members of this Subcommittee, federal and state regulators, medical professionals and the general public, are deeply disturbed by the events we have learned of over the past two months with respect to Peanut Corporation of America (PCA).

These events have had a very significant impact on our consumers and our Company, and we regret any role our products may have played in the Salmonella outbreak. We thank the Subcommittee for the opportunity to discuss these important issues, in particular, how we can work together to strengthen the safety of the U.S. food supply.

PCA'S BUSINESS WITH KELLOGG

PCA's Blakely, Georgia facility was one of our suppliers of peanut paste, that we used in our Cary, North Carolina bakery to manufacture *Austin*® and *Keebler*® brand peanut butter sandwich crackers. PCA also supplied ingredients to other companies that manufacture certain limited product lines for Kellogg. We received our first shipment of peanut paste from PCA in July, 2007.

Consistent with Kellogg protocol, we qualified PCA to do business through our multistep qualification process prior to receiving shipments from them. The initial step in this qualification process is requiring that PCA provide us with an independent, third-party food safety audit report. It is common industry practice to rely on third-party audits to supplement a company's own requirements for suppliers.

PCA provided us with an independent audit report prepared for them in 2006 by American Institute of Baking International (AIB). AIB is one of several audit firms commonly relied on in the food industry. The report gave PCA an "Excellent" rating and noted some minor improvements needed. We requested information from PCA to verify that the improvements were made. PCA provided us with written certification that corrective actions had been taken.

At the same time, we required PCA to complete a risk analysis assessment, which we refer to as our Raw Material Information Sheet (RMIS). This requires a supplier to provide comprehensive information on a variety of factors, including documentation of safety plans (such as Hazard Analysis and Critical Control Point (HACCP)), allergen controls, microbiological parameters and test methodologies). This tool serves as the foundation for our ongoing monitoring of a supplier.

Another step in the process requires suppliers to represent in writing in the form of a "Certificate of Analysis" that an independent lab has confirmed that the ingredient supplied has, among other things, tested negative for pathogens, including *Salmonella*.

As part of our ongoing supplier monitoring, Kellogg also requires qualified suppliers to provide annual independent, audits of their facilities. PCA retained AIB to conduct food safety audits in 2007 and 2008 of their Blakely, Georgia facility. AIB audited core areas of food safety including: "Adequacy of Food Safety Program," "Pest Control," "Operational Methods and Personnel Practices," "Maintenance for Food Safety" and "Cleaning Practices."

Audit findings reported no concerns that the facility may have had any pathogen-related issues or any potential contamination. In fact, each report provided that PCA had formalized programs in place, including a HACCP program, as well as a program for the control of bacteria that included sending environmental samples to outside laboratories for testing. In addition, the reports referenced the results of the plant's most recent regulatory inspections where no, or only a few minor, issues had been found. None of the *Salmonella* or hygiene issues that have been reported by regulators over the past several months were noted in any of the audit reports provided to Kellogg.

KELLOGG'S RESPONSE

On January 12, 2009, PCA advised our Cary facility of an issue with specific peanut butter lots produced in their Blakely, Georgia facility. Kellogg purchased only peanut paste, not peanut butter, from that facility.

On January 13th, the Food & Drug Administration (FDA) notified us that Kellogg's *Austin*® peanut butter sandwich crackers may be implicated in PCA's *Salmonella* problems. We requested information about the specific products, lot dates and Universal Product Codes, and information on whether tested products were open or unopened. Unfortunately, FDA was unable to provide these details.

Despite having very limited information about a possible implication for our products, we immediately activated our Corporate Incident Management Team, a multidisciplinary team that investigates, among other issues, significant quality and food safety issues. The team commenced an internal investigation including reviewing our own environmental pathogen testing results at our Cary facility (the location where peanut butter sandwich crackers are produced), which were all negative for *Salmonella*. We also reviewed the Certificates of Analysis that PCA had provided Kellogg for each lot of paste received, and they were also all negative for *Salmonella*. Despite our findings, and out of an abundance of caution, we shut the lines down that day at our Cary facility and put product shipments on hold.

On January 14, 2009, per Kellogg protocol, the Corporate Incident Management Team briefed my senior management team and me on the situation. Based on the information provided, we made the decision to initiate a "pull and hold" with respect to our *Austin*® and *Keebler*® peanut butter sandwich crackers which contained PCA paste.

This involved two steps. First, we contacted customers that day and instructed them to pull these products from shelves until further notice by Kellogg so that the product would not be available for purchase. Second, we issued a press release advising consumers not to eat previously purchased peanut butter sandwich crackers because of possible risk of *Salmonella* contamination.

Two days later, on January 16, 2009, PCA extended its recall to include limited 2008 lots of peanut paste, plus additional lots of peanut butter. At that time, Kellogg escalated its pull and hold to a voluntary Class I recall of peanut butter cracker sandwiches back to July 1, 2008. We also recalled two snack-pack sized cookies which a co-manufacturer had informed us had been produced using impacted PCA peanut butter lots.

As PCA recalls expanded, Kellogg promptly expanded its recalls of impacted products. In total, more than 7 million cases of our products were recalled due to the PCA contamination at a cost of approximately $ 65-70 million. We devoted significant staffing and resources to quickly trace our products, notify and inform customers and the general public, and execute our recalls to protect our consumers.

Since we first learned of the PCA investigation, Kellogg has worked closely and cooperatively with FDA, the Centers for Disease Control and Prevention (CDC) and local agricultural and health authorities in their investigation of PCA and potentially impacted Kellogg products. We immediately shut down manufacturing lines at our Cary facility which had used the PCA peanut paste, isolated other areas of our plant, and did extensive testing of our facility. It is important to note that all of our environmental tests of the Cary plant before the recall were negative for *Salmonella*. In addition, all of the environmental tests done at the Cary plant in connection with the PCA investigation were negative for Salmonella.

We also worked closely with authorities to conduct a precautionary and extensive hygienic cleaning of all the lines in our plant that used PCA paste. All of the tests run after that hygienic cleaning have been negative for *Salmonella*.

We were deeply disturbed by reports that *Salmonella* was identified in two samples of our peanut butter cracker products. We reached out to the FDA and CDC for more information on those results and continue to cooperate with officials in their ongoing investigations.

Kellogg's Continuous Improvement

The PCA situation has shown that if a company chooses to ignore even basic food safety principles, food safety systems and protections can be compromised, whether those are individual company systems or the U.S. food safety system generally.

Our food safety program operates on the principle that food safety is a process of continuous improvement. In that spirit, and as a result of what we learned from this unfortunate situation, we have taken several immediate actions. We established new cross-functional Kellogg audit teams, including our Quality, Food Safety and Materials Management groups, to audit suppliers of high-risk ingredients, and have already completed on-site audits of our peanut and peanut paste ingredient suppliers. We are requiring suppliers to conduct environmental testing and monitoring in their plants to assist in identifying, assessing and correcting potential contamination before it becomes a food safety problem. We are also strengthening our internal training and education across our supply chain.

Recommendations for Industry Improvements

The recent outbreak illustrated that the U.S. food safety system must be strengthened. We believe the key is to focus on prevention, so that potential sources of contamination are identified and properly addressed before they become actual food safety problems.

Attachment I outlines recommended enhancements which Kellogg believes would enhance the safety of the nation's food supply. You will note that we support several principles: (i) the formation of a single food safety authority under Health and Human Services that will give accountability to one agency leader for science, surveillance, research and inspection, with support from a science-based Food Safety Advisory Council; (ii) a requirement that every food company conduct a risk analysis and document their preventative controls, verification systems and testing results in a food safety plan that is subject to regular FDA review; (iii) annual inspections by FDA of facilities producing high-risk products; (iv) working with industry and government to align around a single food safety standard for evaluating facilities, with appropriate training and accreditation of auditors and auditing firms; and (v) ensuring that FDA has the right mix of intervention and enforcement powers.

Kellogg is firmly committed to working together with Congress, industry and other stakeholders to evaluate and advance these recommendations.

Attachment I : Kellogg Company Recommendations for Enhancements to U.S. Food Safety System

Prevention

Single Food Safety Authority within Health & Human Services (HHS): There is an opportunity to strengthen and maximize the efficiency of regulatory oversight by aligning food safety leadership within HHS. If adequately funded, there is a public health benefit to be gained if a single HHS leader has direct line control over science, research, surveillance and different inspectional units and staffs. This allows HHS to focus food safety resources on products and practices that may contribute to foodborne illness. In addition, a Food Safety Advisory Council comprised of government and industry food safety experts should be established and permanently funded to support development of enhanced science-based food safety policies and standards. We also support the Obama administration's effort to create a new food safety working group to coordinate interagency food safety efforts.

Risk analysis and Food Safety Plans: The production of safe foods starts with prevention, which is accomplished by identifying potential risks in the food production system and developing a proactive plan to prevent or eliminate these risks before they become food safety issues. All food manufacturers should be required to conduct a risk analysis and to develop a food safety plan for FDA review. The plan should document appropriate preventative controls and verification steps. In particular, manufacturers of high-risk foods should be obligated to monitor their manufacturing environments for *Salmonella,* to keep a record of all *Salmonella* positive test results and their corrective actions, and to make these records available during an FDA inspection. By requiring disclosure of positive *Salmonella* test results during inspection, the FDA can assess how the company responded and whether the appropriate corrective actions were taken.

Improve Current Good Manufacturing Practices (GMPs): Stakeholders in food safety have learned much since GMPs were last updated 22 years ago. Congress should mandate a deadline for the agency to update GMPs to reflect new information, particularly in the areas of training, allergen control, control of manufacturing environment (pathogen environmental monitoring) and sanitation.

International Food Protection Training Institute: Kellogg Company supports establishing an "International Food Protection Training Institute" to train government and industry inspectors. This Institute would provide a first-in-class, career spanning curriculum developed and implemented by the Association of Food and Drug Officials (AFDO). Inspectors would be trained to inspect against widely recognized food quality and safety standards to enhance the consistency of inspections.

Intervention

Annual FDA Inspection of Facilities Manufacturing High-Risk Foods: FDA must ensure all companies, big and small, are producing safe products. One way to accomplish this objective is to have all facilities which manufacture high-risk foods inspected regularly. Currently, many of these manufacturing facilities are not inspected on a frequent basis, leaving potential gaps in the overall food safety system. Consequently, we recommend that FDA perform an annual inspection of each high-risk food manufacturing facility.

Food Manufacturing Facility Audit Standard: Food manufacturers, retailers and consumers would benefit from a universal food safety standard for evaluating food manufacturing facilities. The standard should be developed through a transparent and open process. We support efforts to develop this standard and to train, certify and accredit third-party auditors and auditing firms to ensure that audits are conducted in a consistent manner.

Mandatory Recall Authority: Responsible food companies remove foods from the marketplace when there is a concern regarding their safety. Providing the FDA with mandatory recall authority would remove any obstacles that could delay or prevent the removal of potentially unsafe foods from the marketplace.

Response

Traceability of Ingredients: Congress should direct the FDA to work with food manufacturers, farmers and retailers to explore traceability systems, and to explore new technologies that can integrate different traceability systems without abandoning investments made in response to bioterror laws.

In: The Salmonella Outbreak in Peanut Products: The FDA … ISBN: 978-1-60741-950-1
Editor: Benjamin K. Glynn

Chapter 21

SALMONELLA & INDUSTRY ROLE IN PROTECTION HEARING-ISELY TESTIMONY

Heather C. Isely

INTRODUCTION

Good morning, Chairman Stupak, Ranking Member Walden, and Members of the Subcommittee. My name is Heather C. Isely, and I am Executive Vice President and part owner of Vitamin Cottage Natural Food Markets, Inc. We are also known to the communities we serve as Vitamin Cottage,Natural Grocers, or sometimes just The Cottage. I am pleased to be here today with our company s Director of Special Projects, Mr. Alan P. Lewis.

In light of the serious and tragic reasons for this hearing, we very much appreciate the opportunity to provide our input to the subcommittee on our involvement with the Peanut Corporation of America (PCA) and to provide insight on how outbreaks like this one are dealt with by small-chain retailers. We are encouraged by President Obama s recent call for increased food safety and by Chairman Waxman s and this Committees unfailing persistence in improving food safety.

COMPANY HISTORY AND PROFILE

Vitamin Cottage was established in 1955 by my parents, Margaret and Philip Isely. They started the business by going door-to-door in Golden, Colorado, selling whole-grain bread and sharing nutrition information with people they met. Philip and Margaret Isely found that the more health and nutrition knowledge their neighbors possessed, the healthier the food they would buy and eat. Their door-to-door business was successful enough that within a short time they were able to open their first retail location a modest storefront that looked l ke a cottage. Gradually they were able to build their purchasing power to buy at lower cost, which allowed more customers to afford their healthy offerings. To this day, combining nutrition education with affordable, healthy foods drives our business model.

Our business is still privately held and family-owned and operated by my family. Together we strive to carry on my parentsegacy, and fifty-five years after they founded the company the goals of Vitamin Cottage now Natural Grocers remain the same. We focus on providing exceptional customer service, an extensive nutritional and health information service, and the highest quality products at affordable prices.

Natural Grocers has now grown from a tiny "mom and pop" business to a thirty-store chain with over one thousand employees in Colorado, New Mexico, and Texas. Whenever feasible, we add more stores based on the needs of individual communities. Our stores tend to be in the 10,000 square foot range, which is about 1/4 to 1/8 the size of a conventional supermarket. We stock approximately 10,000 carefully selected natural and organic food items, as well as an equally large selection of natural body care items, household goods, and nutritional supplements. We offer a full selection of healthy frozen foods, bulk foods, some cold prepared foods, prepackaged meats, poultry and fish, dairy products, and 100% organic produce. To maintain a scrupulously clean environment for our customers and to keep overhead costs low, we do *not* operate bakeries, butcher shops, cheese shops, hot prepared foods, salad bars, juice bars, coffee bars or other similar food preparation in our stores.

THE RECENT PCA RECALL

For over thirty years, Natural Grocers has offered organic peanut butter for purchase by our customers under its own brandedlabel. We have small grinding machines in our stores into which trained employees place dry roasted peanuts; the peanut butter exits the machine into tubs labeled Vitamin Cottage, which are sealed. I recent years, Natural Grocers has sold about 5,000 pounds of fresh ground peanut butter each month. For the past few years, the dry roasted peanuts purchased for this product have been purchased from PCA. According to paperwork and verbal verification received from the company, all of this peanut stock was produced by PCA in their Plainview, Texas facility. Until the outbreak that is the subject of this hearing, Natural Grocers has never had any health issues associated either with its peanut butter or other private label products.

Beginning in November 2008, the Centers for Disease Control (CDC) identified a suspicious outbreak pattern of *Salmonella serotype Typhimurium* widely dispersed across the country. During their subsequent investigation, in cooperation with the Food and Drug Administration (FDA) and state public health agencies, the CDC linked the growing outbreak to peanut products produced by the PCA facility in Blakely, Georgia. On January 10th, 2009, PCA posted its first recall notice for PCA-made King Nut peanut butter. During January, PCA expanded its recall to all peanut butter products produced in Blakely, but publicly maintained that products from its other two plants were not implicated in the recall. During this time, Natural Grocers received extensive lists of hundreds of recalled products that potentially contained PCA-sourced ingredients. Daily (sometimes hourly), more products were removed from our shelves and recall list updates were posted both in stores and on our company websites. On January 21 of this year, FDA initiated investigations of PCA s Texas and Virginia facilities. Natural Grocers was not notified of this inspection or any negative findings related to this inspection. Despite continuing quality assurances from personnel at the PCA-Texas plant, Natural Grocers quarantined its inventory of PCA peanut products on

January 28th. On January 30th, Natural Grocers voluntarily recalled all unground and ground PCA peanut butter stock, and began notifying customers to return all previously purchased fresh ground peanut butter. On February 10, 2009, the FDA added a Vitamin Cottage fresh ground peanut butter recall notice to its web site.

Epidemiological Link to PCA-Texas Plant

Of the total eighteen confirmed cases of Salmonella in Colorado, two patients presented the Colorado Department of Public Health (CDPH)with especially good data to trace back the outbreak. Based on what information was allowed to be released to us under patient privacy rules, both case-patients were four-year-old children with severe allergies, from different households. Due to the allergies, both families carefully controlled the diet to exclude tree nuts. Natural Grocers fresh ground peanut butter was reported to be one of the few peanut-related products the boys were allowed to consume, since it was a safe, single-ingredient product produced in a nut grinder used exclusively for peanuts. These reports, combined with our confirmation that we used PCA-Texas peanut butter stock in this product, led investigators to conclude that there existed a possible associationbetween these two case patients, our fresh ground peanut butter, and the PCA Texas plant. (Neither of these case-patients was reported hospitalized.)

According to our understanding based on conversations with the CDPH, there have been two hospitalizations of Colorado case-patients; one of these case-patients did not report consuming PCA peanut butter, while the other had eaten some PCA peanut butter along with several other suspect foods.

Of the dozens of peanut and peanut butter samples tested, there are only two positive tests for the outbreak strain of Salmonella. However, these samples are of limited value to the trace- back investigation because the samples were acquired from opened containers taken from households where salmonella was present.

Company Participation with CDC/FDA Trace-Back Investigation

Natural Grocers became one of the primary reference companies of the CDC, FDA, and the CDPH trace-back investigation for a number of reasons:

The company had a long history of using PCA peanuts and maintained a record of lot numbers relevant to the outbreak.

The company sold a large quantity of single-ingredient peanut product, which could help eliminate other ingredients as possible sources of the salmonella contamination. (Most other recalled products used PCA peanut products along with many other ingredients.)

Our retail locations were very well maintained and clean, and we did not allow customers to operate (and therefore potentially contaminate) our peanut butter grinding machines. Trained staff following strict food safety guidelines in grinding the peanuts and cleaning the machines. (This is in stark contracts to other retailers, who allow unsupervised customer access to peanut butter grinders and to the bulk peanut stock.)

Our peanut butter grinders were meticulously maintained and cleaned, so that extensive pathogen testing on the equipment successfully eliminated the machines as potential sources of the salmonella outbreak strain.

We have one grinder in each store dedicated to peanut butter; it is not shared with other products (either intentionally or accidentally by customer usage).

Of the fourteen or so initial confirmed Salmonella cases in our marketing area, six cases reported having PCA peanut butter from Vitamin Cottage in their pantries, and two of these patients were on carefully controlled diets and reported eating only PCA peanut butter as the only potential source of infection.

Natural Grocers was willing and able to fully and proactively support all public health authorities, and dedicated several high-level employees to help the various public health agencies in the trace-back investigation.

We were able to provide hundreds of PCA peanut samples from both sealed and open containers, with associated lot numbers, to FDA inspectors within hours of their request.

Natural Grocers conducted its own extensive testing on unground PCA peanuts, unsold ground PCA peanut butter, and customer-returned PCA peanut butter in early February via federally accredited microbiology laboratories. (100% of these tests were negative for Salmonella; all lab results are included in our documentation previously submitted to the Committee.)

FDA Food Protection Plan

We have carefully reviewed the 2007 FDA Food Protection Plan to see how we can support our government s efforts toward improved food safety. Below is a representative checklist of responsibilities and obligations that will fall to Natural Grocers when an improved food safety system is fully implemented. Please know that we are in full compliance for our part in this shared effort to ensure that American consumers can trust that the food they buy is safe to eat. The FDA Plan, is organized with three principles: Prevention, Intervention, and Response. Here is our current status in regard to compliance with these plans:

PREVENT Food-Borne Contamination

Source food domestically when possible.

Source products and ingredients from known reliable companies who follow current Good Manufacturing Practices.

Maintain food handling facilities that are compliant with US government, state, county and local regulations and guidance.

Continually improve our internal food safety program and share significant advances with industry partners and the government authorities.

Pay special attention to imported foods and be aware of potential criminal or terrorist activity.

Institute sample testing of food products identified as high-risk.

INTERVENE at Critical Points in the Food Supply Chain

Increase quality and frequency of food processing facility inspections.

Assist in education employees and consumers about food-borne illness awareness and prevention at all levels of the food production system.

Assist in educating food producers about food-borne illnesses.

Report possible dangers present at a food processing facilities.

Implement appropriate inspection, tracking, reporting, auditing and training programs.

RESPOND Rapidly to Minimize Harm

Report positive pathogen tests within 24 hours and quarantine product

Maintain adequate and accessible trace-back information beyond the shelf life of a product.

Voluntarily recall potentially contaminated products.

Provide the means to notify consumers within our reach about immediate dangers of potentially contaminated food once we have been notified of them.

Cooperate with all investigations related to food borne illnesses.

Allow emergency access to certain records and facilities related to a potential food safety threat.

We are proud to report to the Committee today that Natural Grocers is substantially compliant with key elements of the proposed Food Safety plan.

Affect of Proposed FDA Food Safety System on the Current Salmonella Outbreak

According to reports, PCA was able to operate under the radarof local, state and federal regulatory agencies while disregarding even basic food safety procedures. We agree with the FDA that the burden should be placed on private industry to develop and implement comprehensive food safety requirements as needed for their particular situation, equipment, foodstuffs and type of processing. We also agree that highly competent and empowered third party inspection and audit teams would probably have discovered, reported, and corrected alleged PCA violations and potentially avoided the current Salmonella outbreak. And we agree that at very least, a legal requirement to report positive pathogen results and destroy contaminated product, if complied with, would have at least limited the scope of the outbreak. Natural Grocers relied on PCA s representations of compliance with Good Manufacturing Practices, its certificate of compliance with the National Organic Program from an USDA accredited agency (the highly respected Texas Dept of Agriculture) and other information to determine that PCA s products were safe for consumption. However, a number of competent individuals whether inside the plant, with government agencies, or with private companies -- appear to have had knowledge of material violations of food safety practices at PCA plants, yet failed to intervene.

Peanuts, until recently, have generally not been considered high risk for Salmonella contamination and would not have been subject to sampling and testing at the retail level under FDA risk assessment guidelines. Subsequent to this outbreak, we are sample testing each lot of peanut butter stock from our new supplier. Stock will not be released` for use unless all tests come back negative.

As part of our existing internal food-borne illness alert system, we encourage our customers to report any possible bad health affects they suspect may be caused by the food we sell. We have received notice from three customers during the four months of this outbreak who stated they became ill with various gastrointestinal complaints, and had in the prior days consumed PCA peanut butter among many other foods. (The CDPH was informed verbally of these three reports.) After our store staff record the customersnformation, our Home Office staff contacts the customer for follow up if they have provided contact information. It is our opinion that given the information in these reports there would have been no reporting requirement under the proposed rules, because there was no confirmation possible via lab test, and the cases were unrelated in time, location, symptoms or duration of illness. Had these reports contained critical events, we would have asked the consumer to contact the FDA district office to make a formal consumer food-borne illness complaint. These reports are included in our responsive documents, and we would welcome guidance from the Committee on our responsibilities associated with them.

Our Approach to Food Safety

Natural Grocers was founded in 1955 for the sole purposed of improving our family s and our neighbors health through better nutrition using a wholesome balanced diet. This was at a time when a good working knowledge of nutrition was quite rare, and when highly processed foods with many questionable ingredients filled the shelves of most stores. Please see our website s statement on *What We Don t Sell and Why*–our first line of defense in regard to food safety is not to allow potentially dangerous substances into the foods we sell. Some of these substances are more immediately dangerous than others; however, when you keep other families as loyal customers over four generations, like we have, the subtle long term cumulative affects of even minute amounts of risky substances really, really matters. As a guiding principle, we will not sell a product today if it means possibly causing someone harm at any time in the future.

In addition to setting very high standards for the products we sell, we also set very high standards for the companies from which we buy. For each of the quality products on our shelves, it is certainly possible to find a much less expensive stand-in that might sell just as well but not really have the same nutritional value or meet our clean food standards. We only work with companies that have rigorous and transparent quality control standards. For critical categories such as meat and poultry, we personally inspect the operations and monitor their compliance with our own set of standards. These inspections are in addition to all of the health department and USDA protocols already in place.

Comprehensive Science-Based Approach to Nutrition and Food Safety

Our approach to food safety often puts us out ahead of government. We are often in the position of educating customers about why our safety standards are much more broad and strict than the government's.

When new research is published, we as a company proactively deal with potentially dangerous or unhealthy products. The government regulatory process is much more complicated–it has to encompass the values and concerns of hundreds of millions of constituents, many of whom have irreconcilable views. I will share a few examples of how Natural Grocers has already responded well in advance of new government rules being issued, based on the generally accepted conclusions of the scientific community.

The reason our internal food safety standards often exceed government standards is that as a private company we can approach food safety with a different starting question. We ask Might this Substance do Harm?. This is a significantly different approach than required of public health authorities, who start by asking if an ingredient is Generally Recognized As Safe. To be clear, we understand why legislators and regulators take a different approach to clearing new foods or medicines, and we are not criticizing that approach or suggesting it be modified. We would agree that one of the government s roles as the delegated representative of the common good is to prevent harm being done to the whole by any one individual's (or corporation's) acts. Nevertheless, when the government cannot demonstrate harm being done by a substance, it is unlikely to have cause to promulgate regulations.

While Natural Grocers fully supports and complies with this approach to creating policy that protects the public, we operate our business on behalf of a constituency that asks for a more stringent standard of protection. Clearly, our company s offerings do *not* appeal to everyone. To illustrate this point, try imagining the grocery store where you shop: it is probably almost as big as a football field with row upon row of processed packaged goods lined up every three yards between the end zones and sidelines. In the stands surrounding the field are produce, dairy products, a deli, a meat and a fish counter. Now, imagine that store without any products that contain artificial colorings or preservatives. If you are doing this exercise right, all those shelves on the turf just lost most all of their products. Now take away dairy and animal products created with added growth hormones and antibiotics and take away produce grown with non-organic pesticides, herbicides, and cleaners (or co-mingled with produce that was). By now you should have in your mind s eye a huge empty stadium with row after row of empty seats, empty shelves, empty dairy cases, and empty produce aisles.

Natural Grocers will not sell just anything to turn a profit.. And for good reason, because our core customers, many of whom encounter difficulty shopping anywhere else, rely on us. Consider:

Customers with severe gluten allergies prefer to shop where there is no gluten contamination in the air from an in-store bakery;

Customers with compromised immune systems due to chronic illness or chemotherapy require almost sterile conditions to stay well. This is very difficult to accomplish with butcher shops and delis on site;

Customers hypersensitive to odors can become nauseated in a conventional grocery. We do not waft heavy scents through our stores via cooking or artificially improvedhousehold goods;

Customers who are uncomfortable with animal blood and carcasses appreciate not seeing or smelling fish and animal carcasses on display. We buy only pre-packaged meat, poultry and fish;

Customers sensitive to the harsh chemicals found in conventional household items feel safer knowing our products are selected with their needs in mind; and,

Customers who are vigilant parents of young children, or vigilant children of aging parents, who trust that we only stock foods that are good, clean, and safe for their vulnerable loved ones to consume.

For every potential customer who is unhappy that we wont sell them Tide Ultra detergent, just-baked sweet rolls or bowls of seafood medley, there is another that is very happy that we dont. Another very important reason for avoiding store-prepared foods is that they tend to increase the cost of food while decreasing its nutritional value. Since our customers are often focused on the principles of clean food and good nutrition, and, tend to be quite frugal, our offerings lean toward simple, natural ingredients. Healthy food does no good if you cant afford to buy it.

CONCLUSION

Again, I appreciate the opportunity to testify before the Subcommittee, and welcome any questions you may have.

In: The Salmonella Outbreak in Peanut Products: The FDA … ISBN: 978-1-60741-950-1
Editor: Benjamin K. Glynn

Chapter 22

SALMONELLA & INDUSTRY ROLE IN PROTECTION HEARING-LIGHTSEY EMAIL

Sammy Lightsey

From: "Sammy Lightsey" peanutcorp.com>
To: "'Pete Hatfield'" aibonline.org>
Date: 12/31/2008 9:45 AM
Subject:, RE: Greetings//19408/19408-A
We will only have one audit and March 23 and 24 is good.

—Original Message--
From: Pete Hatfield aibonline.org]
Sent Monday, December , : 8 PM
To: Sammy Lightsey
Cc: Jermaine Dillon; Peg Ray
Subject RE: Greetings//19408/19408-A

Hi Sammy,

Are you going to stay with the two different audits like in the past?? If so, then your audits will take at least 1.5 days, maybe two, since we have a new audit format to work from.

As far as someone for QA Manager, I am sure you know more qualified people than I do.

I am scheduling you for audit dates on March 23 and 24, Monday and Tuesday. Let me know if these are acceptable.

Pete

>>> "Sammy Lightsey" peanutcorp.com> 12/29/2008 12:52 PM >>>

Hello Pete,

Yes, We did get the new standards. I am in the process of hiring a new QA Manager and would like to a little time to bring him or her up to speed. Would you have any idea of anyone that may be interested in the job. Let's schedule February 23rd and 24th or maybe sometime in March. Thanks and I look forward with working with you again.

Sammy

---Original Message--
From: Pete Hatfield /aibonline.org]
Sent Monday, December 22, 2008 10:55 AM
To: sammy.lightsey
Subject Greetings

Hello again Sammy Lightsey,

You lucky guy, I am your AIB auditor. So we need to get your plant set up for any audit Please be informed first off that we are using a new standard. I am assuming that you have received an updated copy of the AIB Food Safety Standards. I am also assuming that you have or will review and will note the changes you need to make in order not to have points deducted when we do the audit. If not, let me know.

Secondly, we need to schedule your audit. It looks like your plant will require 1.5 days to complete the two audits using the new formats. Rather than the one day we used in the past.

Looking at this from a 1.5 day audit setup, I have these dates available, you let me know which one will work best for you. I have January 6, 7 and 8 open. I have February 10, 11, 12 and 13 open. I have February 23 and 24 open.

Please try to pick from these dates. Hopefully you will pick the earliest date possible.

If you wish to talk, call me at home, .cell phone or home

Thanks and Merry Christmas and Happy New Year to you and your family,

Pete Hatfield

In: The Salmonella Outbreak in Peanut Products: The FDA … ISBN: 978-1-60741-950-1
Editor: Benjamin K. Glynn

Chapter 23

SALMONELLA & INDUSTRY ROLE IN PROTECTION HEARING-SLAWINSKI EMAIL

Tim Slawinski

From: Slawinski, Tim
Sent: Thursday, February 5, 2009 10:00 AM
To: Tong, Jennifer
Cc: Chestnut, Tom Bail, James
Subject: RE: AIB named at Peanut Corp

Yeah. However, if the FDA sent their team of inspectors to the facility before the outbreak occurred with no knowledge of whether there was a problem at the facility or not, would they really have found these problems? I'm pretty confident they would have had similar results as the State of Georgia and the multiple third party firms that inspected the place. Plus, the biggest problem was with the positive micro data that they ignored. From my understanding, this data was not initially available for the FDA either. They had to really pry into their documentation before uncovering the additiohal test results. The media may not understand the difference between a full blown FDA investigation and a routine inspection, but I'm hoping the FDA does.

Tim Slawinski
Assistant Director
Food Safety & Quality
NSF International
Phone:
Fax:

----Original Message-----
From: Tong, Jennifer
Sent: Thursday, February 05, 2009 9:10 AM

To: Slawinski, Tim
Cc: Chestnut, Tom; Bail, James
Subject: RE: AIB named at Peanut Corp

Not good for auditing companies in general as we work with the FDA to try to get them to recognize 3rd party inspection/certification in lieu of government oversight.

Jen

From: Slawinski, Tim
Sent: Wednesday, February 04, 2009 11:52 PM
To: Bail, James; Chestnut, Tom; Tong, Jennifer
Subject: AIB named at Peanut Corp

FYI. New York Times article names AIB as one of the third party companies at Peanut Corp.
Peanut Plant Says Audits Declared It in Top Shape

By *ANDREW MARTIN*
Published: February 4, 2009

A company at the center of a huge and deadly *salmonella* outbreak said Wednesday that its peanut plant was regularly visited last year by private inspectors, several of whom declared it to be in tip-top shape.

In a statement released Wednesday, the company, Peanut Corporation of America, reported "regular visits and inspections" of its Blakely, Ga., plant in 2008, not only by federal and state regulators but by independent auditors and *food safety* companies that made "customary unannounced inspections."

At least one of the private inspectors was hired by the peanut company itself, which provided the audit to customers to meet their food safety requirements.

One of the private inspectors "gave the plant an overall superior rating," the peanut company's statement said. "The other rated the plant as 'meets or exceeds audit expectations (Acceptable-Excellent) ratings.' "

Peanut Corporation of America's statement was released as food manufacturers and public health officials tried to determine how so many inspectors missed what some have said were obvious problems at the plant, including improper sanitation procedures, live roaches, mold and slimy residue on floors and equipment.

Federal officials have begun a criminal inquiry of the peanut company after learning that it knowingly shipped products that had tested positive for salmonella. The outbreak has caused more than 500 illnesses and eight deaths. More than 1,000 products have been recalled, including pet food, ice cream and brownies.

Kellogg, one of the companies that recalled peanut products, received reports of third-party independent audits of Peanut Corporation of America in 2007 and 2008. The audits, paid for by the peanut company to meet food manufacturers' requirements, were intended to. assess its compliance with federally mandated manufacturing practices, including the condition of the plant and equipment and cleanliness, said Kris Charles, a spokeswoman for Kellogg.

Audits are also supposed to review the supplier's food safety program, microbial test results and internal audit results.

Each audit, conducted by AIB International, gave the Blakely plant a "superior" rating. "We are looking into whether the third-party auditor reviewed state inspection reports or the plant's test results," Ms. Charles said by "It is certainly something we would have expected them to do because it is an audit requirement." Kellogg also received written test results from Peanut Corporation of America that the peanut paste it had supplied Kellogg showed no positive salmonella results, she said.

Had Kellogg known of the problems at the plant that the *Food and Druq Administration* detailed recently, "we would have discontinued the relationship with P.C.A. immediately and would not have accepted any ingredients from them," she said.

Jim Munyon, president of AIB International, based in Manhattan, Kan., said he Could not release details of the peanut company's audit because of confidentiality agreements. He said the company would not have received a superior rating if his auditors had seen the filth the federal government described.

"It would mean that we didn't see it on the day we were there," he said of the rating. "What goes on the rest of the time, we don't know."

He said his company relies on his customers to provide details of internal microbial tests. Had the peanut company divulged the presence of salmonella, he said, "We would have had a discussion about those failures."

Doug Powell, an associate professor of food safety at *Kansas State University,* said the salmonella outbreak at Peanut Corporation of America showed the "fallacy" of independent audits, which are commonly used to verify food safety, animal welfare claims and organic production methods. While the intent might be good, he said, the results are usually withheld from the public.

"Companies say they do all this testing. Great. Show us.the data. They won't," Mr. Powell said. "Given all the outbreaks, why should we believe them?"

In: The Salmonella Outbreak in Peanut Products: The FDA … ISBN: 978-1-60741-950-1
Editor: Benjamin K. Glynn

Chapter 24

SALMONELLA & INDUSTRY ROLE IN PROTECTION HEARING- NESTLÉ 2006 AUDIT

Nestlé North America

Nestlé North America Nestlé

ATE: January 15, 2006

TO: [redacted], North York, Purchasing
[redacted] Glendale, Purchasing
[redacted] Director Quality Management, Prepared Foods Division
[redacted] Manager, Division Quality Management
[redacted] North York, Ice Cream
[redacted] London, Quality Assurance

CC: [redacted] Director Central Audit
[redacted] Central Audit T & P Specialist

Audit Team Members
Other Auditor(s)

Peanut Corporation of America
Stewart Parnell, President
Stewart Adams, Technical Director
Danny Kilgore, S.E. Operations Manager
Jim Booher, Plant Manager
Stan Januta, QC Manager

From:	[redacted]@us.nestle.com
Audit Type:	NQS Level 1 – Food Safety Audit Report
Name of Facility:	Peanut Corporation of America
Audit Date:	January 5, 2006

From:	[redacted]@us.nestle.com
Audit Type:	NQS Level 1 – Food Safety Audit Report
Name of Facility:	Peanut Corporation of America
Audit Date:	January 5, 2006

Holding Company:	Peanut Corporation of America	
Address:	PO Box 10037 Lynchburg, Virginia 24506	Phone: [redacted] FAX #: [redacted]

Facility Type:	Raw Material Supplier	
Address:	3601 North I-27 Plainview, Texas 79072	Phone: [redacted] FAX #: (xxx) xxx-xxxx
☐ Other locations manufacturing for Nestlé. [Reference Supplier Co-manufacturer Quality Survey]		
Status:	☐ Active	☒ Potential

Nestlé Factory Locations Supplied:	London		
Product(s):	Diced or granulated peanuts		
Application(s):	Drumstick Ball Top Cones		
Risk Level Assigned:	High		
Nestlé Businesses:	**Nestlé USA:** ☐ Beverage ☐ Confection & Snacks ☐ PetCare ☐ Prepared Foods ☐ Food Services ☐ Nutrition ☐ Foreign Trade ☐ Nestlé-USA Distribution Co	**Nestlé Canada:** ☐ Beverage ☐ Confection & Snacks ☐ PetCare ☒ Prepared Foods ☐ Food Services ☐ Nutrition ☐ Foreign Trade ☐ Nestlé-USA Distribution Co	**Other Market (s):** List the other Nestlé Markets supplied by this facility. ☐ Beverage ☐ Confection & Snacks ☐ PetCare ☐ Prepared Foods ☐ Food Services ☐ Nutrition ☐ Foreign Trade ☐ Nestlé-USA Distribution Co

Final Assessment

	Complying	Complying with Major Improvement Needed	Not Complying
NQS Level 1 – Food Safety	☐	☐ Improvement required within __days.	☐ Disqualified Manufacture of Nestlé product / material is suspended until corrective action measures have been fully implemented, and verified by Nestlé.
Corrective Action / Follow-up Plan Due Date:	Facility is not approved at this time. Response to concerns noted with action plans and timetable should be sent to Dennis Cline by February 10, 2006		

NQS Audit Conclusia

An audit of the Peanut Corporation of America (PCA) facility, in Plainview, Texas was completed on January 5, 2006. The facility does not currently meet NQS Level 1 requirements and would not be qualified from a plant audit standpoint to supply chopped peanut pieces to Nestlé. It was communicated to PCA that a follow up audit by Nestlé would be necessary to verify completion of items requested needing corrective actions.

The key food safety issues noted during this audit are the weakness of the pest control program, the lack of any pathogen environmental monitoring program, and concerns noted in the handling raw and further processed (roasted, blanched) peanuts in a common processing area. Without physical isolation and proper airflow for the post-roasted and roasted peanut operations, there is a potential for microbiological cross contamination.

The audit conditions and deficiencies are outlined in the Key Findings and Key Issues Summary sections of this report. PCA management expressed an understanding and recognition of identified issues, and agreed that each item needed to be brought to closure as soon as possible. It is noted that the gaps identified in the audit should be relatively easy for PCA personnel to resolve and none are beyond their capability to resolve. None of the items identified would require significant capital investment to resolve. It is requested that the facility respond in writing to this report within the timetable as listed below. The response should address all issues identified in the Key Findings and Key issues Summary of this report. The response must address the root cause, identify corrective actions, and provide timelines for correction. The plant is asked to complete the "NQS Audit Corrective Action Response or CAR" Excel spreadsheet at the end of this report and send electronically to the auditor per the above timetable.

It appears as if PCA employees and management have an understanding and commitment to quality, food safety, and customer satisfaction. Plant management staff was very open and cooperative during the audit and expressed a desire to 'iork with customers such as Nestlé to meet expectations.

IQS Level 1 Food Safety Elements	Complying	Complying with Major Improvement Needed	Not Complying
Training	☒		
Documentation	☒		
GMP – Housekeeping	☒		
GMP – Sanitation	☒		
GMP – Pest Control			☒
GMP – Other		☒	
Allergen	☒		
Bio-Security		☒	
HACCP		☒	
QMS	☒		
Pathogen Monitoring of the Production Environment			☒
Formal Release / Status Control System		☒	
Lot Traceability, Lot Identification, Coding / Recall & Crisis Management		☒	
Instrument Calibration / Laboratories and Test Method		☒	

Background Information

Size of Facility:	About 48,000 square feet	Number of employees:	About 35
Age of Facility:	About 45 years	Number of production lines:	1

A Nestlé Quality System Level 1 audit was conducted at the Peanut Corporation of America (PCA), facility in Plainview, Texas, on January 5, 2006 by Dennis Cline. Stewart Parnell, President, Stewart Adams, Technical Director, Danny Kilgore S.E. Operations Manager, Jim Booher, Plant Manager, and Stan Januta, QC Manager, accompanied the auditor throughout the audit.

The purpose of this audit was potential qualification of the Plainview facility to supply chopped roasted peanut pieces initially to the Nestlé London plant, and then eventually to other Nestlé facilities. The Plainview facility consists of a shelled peanut receiving operation whose end product is dry roasted chopped peanut pieces or blanched peanut pieces for the institutional domestic markets. For the purposes of this audit, the entire facility and operation were audited were reviewed.

PCA is part of the Peanut Corporation of America company, Lynchburg, Virginia, and currently supplies peanut products produced in one of three plants (Tidewater, Virginia, Blakely, Georgia, and Plainview, Texas) to the domestic industrial and retail markets.

PCA has supplied product to Nestlé in the past with product processed in the Blakely, Georgia facility, the Plainview facility was originally constructed in the late 1960's and operated as a Jimmy Dean hog slaughter and processing operation. The facility was later sold to the Sara Lee Company, and then Bean Time (pinto bean processor), and then sat idle for about 5 years until PCA purchased the building and property and began renovations just over 1 year ago. Microbiological and environmental studies were conducted in the building and the grounds as part of the purchase negotiation requirements by PCA. The results of these studies were not reviewed as part of this audit, but it was understood that there were no issues noted. The facility is located in Plainview, Texas, a rural area about 40 miles north of Lubbock, Texas. There is easy access to major highway from this location. The plant currently processes on a 16 hour 5 to 6 days a week schedule. Cleaning operations are conducted during the non-processing hours. The plant only processes roasted and / or blanched peanut products,

The facility has been inspected by the Texas Department of Agriculture (TDA) for organic certification, United States Department of Agriculture (USDA) for blancher approval, and kosher. There have been no independent 3rd party audits of this facility.

The general processing steps for processing of dry roasted chopped peanut pieces are below. Shelled peanuts, which are primarily grown in the local southwest region, are received from one of two shellers (Golden or Birdsong). Peanuts are received via truck in 100# burlap bags, cardboard totes, or supersacks. It was understood that the receiving containers were all one-way containers and they are not returned to the shellers to be re-filled.

1. Shelled peanuts are received (supersacks, cardboard totes, or 100# burlap bags)
2. Destoning (Roka de-stoner system)
3. Holding bins
4. Dry roasting (oven) — used if roasting (Aeroglide oven system)
5. Blanching — skin removal
6. Sorting (optical sorting using Sortex 9000)
7. Inspection (visual)
8. Sizing / fines removal
9. Metal detection
10. Pack off into super sacks if for granulation product
11 Short term storage

If granulated, then next steps apply

12. Holding bins
13. Granulation / chopping
14. Sizing
15. Fines removal

16. Packaging
17. Case Metal detection (not yet installed)
18. Palletizing
19. Storage
20. Distribution

There are currently no specifications for products produced for Nestlé. The plant does have PCA specifications for all products produced.

This auditor would like to thank the facility for their cooperation and positive attitude displayed throughout the audit.

TRAINING

Complying

Although training practices are in place, there is no overall documented written training plan, which summarizes the training programs and plant training requirements. A formal written training plan containing plant / company training requirements should be written.

New employee training includes Good Manufacturing Practices (GMP) (program reviewed was dated December 29, 2005), general and job related safety, general HACCP, general allergen, product sampling, and basic plant security information. To acknowledge attendance and participation in training session, each employee and the trainer sign off on a form after the training has been completed.

The GMP training includes hygiene, sanitation; process, and product integrity; receiving and shipping areas; food security; training; and record retention. Training is conducted using video and verbal presentations, and GMP training is conducted in English. All records reviewed in regards to training indicated that the company is following the established procedures.

A temporary employee-training program is followed for the training of any temporary prior to working in the plant. Temporary employees are trained on the same Good Manufacturing Practices as regular full-time plant personal. The temporary employees sign off on a sheet indicating they completed the training.

On going training consists of monthly meeting where topics about GMP and safety are reviewed (same as new hire training). The management team also discusses any incidents / concerns that may have occurred at the plant as a means of continuous improvement.

It is recommended that the plant implement a process by which learning effectiveness is measured. This can be completed by use of short tests following each training session.

Contractors are given GMP and general safety training before entering the plant. The plant GMP and safety rules are reviewed prior to entering the manufacturing areas and a sign off sheet agreeing to these is completed. Contractors, depending on their role, may not be escorted while on site (pest control operator, vending machines, etc.), but all contractors are monitored while on site.

Quality control employees and operators using laboratory equipment are given specific training on how to operate the test equipment.

Overall, employees receive about 8 hours of training annually, with training being spread out over the year. The training starts as a newly hired employee joins the company and continues throughout their employment. The information used for training was reviewed and found to contain sufficient information needed to adequately training employees on safe food handling techniques. All documents and information reviewed was current through today's date.

Employees observed were following the plant established GMP's.

Documentation

Complying

The following documentation was reviewed: employee training, manufacturing guidelines and specifications, plant quality manual, HACCP plan, operating procedures, hold guidelines, receiving / shipping inspection forms, processing checklists, lab equipment calibration records, inspection checklists, start up checklists, pest control service log and schematics, recall program, master sanitation program, sanitation procedures, traceability guidelines, and glass and brittle plastics policy. Documents exist for recording processing and quality checks completed during processing.

A glass and brittle plastics control policy is documented (dated December 29, 2005). It includes requirements for glass and brittle plastics. The program includes procedures for the shielding and protection of light bulbs as well as the exclusion of glass in the plant, an inventory of glass and brittle plastics, and a daily audit of these same items. This procedure clearly defines cleaning and inspection requirements for broken glass incidents.

A customer complaint procedure is documented (dated December 29, 2005). The president, operations manager, and quality manager review complaint issues.

The plant has a document control practice with most all documents being maintained in a paper format. There is no formal written document control procedure. Each document is titled, numbered, and has a date of issue. Most all documentation has been taken from the sister plant in Blakely, Georgia, and is being adjusted to meet the needs of the Plainview facility. The Plant Manager is the final authority for approval of all documents. It was understood that all documents in the document control program are reviewed at least one time per year. An effort needs to be made to make the final transitions of documentation to meet the needs of the local plant.

The plant should create a written Change Management policy that defines steps to be followed for changes that might take place in manufacturing and documentation.

Forms used to record processing conditions and quality data are also included in the document control system and are used on the production floor as paper copies. These documents are collected following processing and are stored in the quality control or accounting office. These forms are reviewed during and after processing by the production supervision and quality management. All forms reviewed during this audit were found to be in the designated format and were current. Good documentation practices were being followed to complete the forms. For each document and form reviewed, there were no cross outs, no scratch outs or re-writes, no pencil usage on the production floor, and no pre-completed information. Pencils were being utilized in the quality control areas. The facility should put forth an effort to eliminate pencils and use blue or black pens in all areas. The processing and quality data is reviewed during and after operations by production and quality personnel.

All documents reviewed were easy to understand, well formatted, and are utilized by the workforce. Plant personnel followed good documentation practices. A copy of the recently developed quality / food safety manual was given to this auditor.

The processing paperwork reviewed in the plant was complete and satisfactory. The records are current through today's date.

GMPs — Housekeeping

Complying With Major Improvement Needed

There was no housekeeping issues noted in the receiving / shipping, processing, chopping / packaging, and storage areas of the plant. There were small amounts of peanut pieces along the south wall and behind electrical panels in the re-clean room. The chemical storage room, maintenance shop, immediate exterior areas around the north and east sides of the plant, employee break room, and bathrooms were also clean and organized.

The exterior areas on the south and west sides of the plant had large amount of dirt and product debris (skins) scattered in depths for about $^{1}/4$ inch to about 8 inches.

There is a remote building on the north side of the plant, which contains what appears to be excess equipment and items removed from the plant. There is a large amount of items stored in piles on the ground. This creates potential harborage areas for insects, rodents, and birds. The building on the southwest corner of the plant used to park the skins collection trailer has unacceptable amounts of product skins accumulated on the floor areas.

Food contact tools and non-food contact tools were separated and appropriately maintained. A number of brooms and shovels have wooden handles. Any tools with wooden handles in the manufacturing areas of the plant should be replaced with non-wooden handled items.

Employees were continually sweeping the floor areas around equipment as needed during the audit.

All packaging materials (cartons, totes, liners, etc.) were covered as appropriate and stored in a designated warehouse area. All items observed stored in the warehouse areas (ambient) were stored on pallets in floor locations.

There was no idle equipment stored in the warehouse areas of the plant.

There was a designated perimeter painted white about 18 inches wide maintained around the warehouse areas. This perimeter was free and clear of product storage, equipment storage, and any other unwanted dirt or debris. Along the exterior southwest wall of the pre-clean room, the concrete at the floor / wall juncture is eroded to a depth of 1 to 2 inches. This area was collecting dirt and debris and is not readily cleanable.

Brooms and other cleaning tools were observed stored hanging on designated racks in designated areas when not in use.

The plant GMPs state that food, beverage, gum, and tobacco products are acceptable in designated areas and are not allowed in the processing and / or warehouse areas of the plant. There were no food, beverage, gum or tobacco items observed in any areas of the plant other than the designated area observed.

There are hand-sanitizing stations located at the entryways to the production areas.

GMPs — Sanitation

Complying

The general overall sanitary condition of the interior of the plant was good. There was minimal product build up on the overhead piping and walls in the pre-clean room. Any product accumulation provides a good environment for potential food source and harborage areas for pests, and a potential foreign material source for any product or equipment that might be located below it when it sloughs off.

The plant is both dry and wet cleaned. Hand tools, brooms, etc., and portable vacuums are used in the facility for some of the dry cleaning requirements. Sanitizer is applied for food contact surfaces after dry cleaning. For wet cleaning, there are no CIP systems in this facility. Some equipment is disassembled and washed in a COP tank.

The plant has established basic cleaning procedures and instructions for the pieces of equipment in the operation. These procedures are developed only for the major tasks. The cleaning standard operating procedures (SOPs) need to be developed throughout the plant to address all wet and dry cleaning. SOPs should be written to outline each task, the cleaning frequency, who is responsible for cleaning, chemicals to be used, chemical concentrations, personal protective equipment, tools needed to complete the task, and anything other information the plant personnel might need for these tasks.

The Master Cleaning Schedule is very basic, and does not include a number of items in the plant such as walls, ceilings, air vents, electrical panels, floor drains, etc. All exterior areas of the plant should be added to master cleaning schedules as poor conditions can lead to potential infestations issues. All of these items should also have procedures developed as described above.

The plant maintains a pre-operational inspection of the processing lines and equipment to assure cleanliness and functionality. Equipment operators are responsible for the sanitation of the equipment they operate. Production supervisors and operators are responsible for ensuring equipment is clean and properly set up prior to start-up.

There are no bulk chemicals for cleaning received at this site.

janitorial supplies are on hand for cleaning the office area and facility restrooms. These are stored in a designated location away from the production areas.

Overall, good sanitation was evident throughout the interior of the facility.

GMPs — Pest Control

Not Complying

The facility uses a 3rd party pest control service — Mcllroy's Pest Control — for pest control services. The plant has a basic pest control policy (dated December 29, 2005) around which the 3rd party program is designed. There is a pest control manual in which the business license, PCO certification, device schematics, services reports, and MSDS sheets are contained. There is no written description of the service that Mcllroy's is to provide. Mcllroy provides service every 2 weeks. All pest control devices are inspected each service. The frequency of device inspection may be increased if determined necessary. A site map, service reports with general or vague inspection comments, PCO certification, company business license, and chemical MSDS sheets are all in order and current. The plant quality control manager is the primary contact for the pest control operator, before, during, and following each service call.

The pest control operator (PCO) is certified in Texas, and has license number 22365 PTLW, which expires March 23, 2006.

The pest control program is supplemented by an in-house warehouse-fogging program utilized during the warmer season. This program consists of routine fogging of the plant warehouse areas utilizing a central system applying Entech Fog 5 (pyrethrum). This pesticide is stored in a locked cage within the maintenance shop. This locked cage area also contains some maintenance items. The pesticide storage area needs to be separated from a routine maintenance use and storage area.

The plant utilizes 36 multi-catch traps (and glue boards) on the interior of the building, and 36 rodent bait stations on the exterior of the building. Pheromone monitors are utilized for stored product pests in the warehouse areas of the plant during the warmer season. Each device is inspected by the PCO during the site visit. All results are documented on the service reports. The plant should work with the PCO to develop a sheet that documents pest activity in a manner that trends can easily be seen. The sheets should be able to easily indicate problem areas or areas of concerns.

The pest control logs for the past 10 months were reviewed with varying levels of rodent activity noted on every report. The activity was primarily noted on the exterior of the building, but there were also concerns in the interior areas of the building. The pest control reports indicate that the plant has an on-going concern with rodent activity occurring at varying levels. The number of devices originally utilized in the service program were doubled after about 5 months of service. The service reports reviewed also say, "seal all voids around doors to prevent pest entry", without noting for which door is a concern. The PCO has utilized a straight line out to indicate some of the devices are being inspected. Each and every device that is inspected should be marked on the log sheet with an individual mark.

The plant maintains asphalt / concrete perimeter on all sides of the building. This area was completely clear except for the pest control devices that had been installed, and the dirt and product debris referenced in the sanitation section above. The paved portions of the property around surrounded by vacant fields. The fields currently contained minimal vegetation and dirt.

During the audit of the exterior of the building, the following was observed:

1. A bait box on north side of building near ramp was missing the top. The rodenticide was on the ground about 2 feet from the stations. There was another bait station installed about 4 feet away from the damaged bait station.
2. The partition walls around the exterior compressor room on the south west corner of the building are constructed of 2 layers of metal with about 3 inches of space in-between the layers. The area inside of this wall was easy viewed (due to the way they had been cut off) contained about 8 to 10 inches of dirt, product debris (skins), and mice carcasses.
3. Mouse carcass lying near bait station #10.
4. 3 mice carcasses and burrows under the grating located near on the wall near the shipping doors.
5. 3 mice carcasses in varying stages of decay lying near bait station #11.
6. 4 mice carcasses in varying stages of decay lying near bait station #12.
7. > 14 mice carcasses in varying stages of decay lying near bait station #13.
8. 5 mice carcasses in varying stages of decay lying near bait station #14.
9. > 10 mice carcasses in varying stages of decay lying near bait station #15.
10. 1 mice carcass in varying stages of decay lying near bait station #18.
11. 3 mice carcasses and 1 rat carcass in varying stages of decay lying near bait station #20.
12. 5 mice carcasses and 1 rat carcass in varying stages of decay lying near bait station #21.
13. 1 mouse carcass in the foam insulation near the corner of the building (area near emergency exit door on the south wall for the pre-clean room).
14. Numerous burrows along area on south side of plant where asphalt ends and dirt begin.
15. A dead pigeon was lying on the ground near the peanut-receiving door.
16. 4 pigeons roosting on the iron support structure inside the skin collection building. The doors to this outside building where hanging open, as the trailer was not completely backed into the building. Based on the feces observed, and by building design, it appears as if bird activity is a problem (and a potential problem) for this building.
17. A lot rodenticide was scattered loosely on the ground on the south and southwest exterior of the building.

There were no insects or rodent activity observed in the interior areas of the plant during the audit.

From my observations during the audit walk through and from the pest control program records, plant management needs to review and revise the current program to incorporate more Integrated Pest Management techniques. This plant has a serious on-going problem with rodents on the exterior portions of the building must be resolved. Although there were no observations of rodents or rodent activity in the interior of the plant noted during this audit, the levels of dead rodents observed, coupled with voids noted around some doorways, indicate there are potential concerns for the interior areas of the plants.

Overall, the current pest control program appears to be less than effective and is unacceptable.

GMPs – Other

Complying with Major Improvement Needed

All areas of the plant observed are in age appropriate condition and maintained in an acceptable manner. Floors (concrete), walls (concrete / metal siding) and ceilings (drop, concrete, metal) were mostly in good repair, with no major cracking or breaks noted. There were no open holes observed in the walls or floors from previous installations, however there were several pipe penetrations through interior walls in the pre-clean room that had not yet been sealed around. Some of the concrete flooring was cracked and broken. This was in particularly poor condition were previous existing walls had been removed. The concrete at the floor / wall juncture on the west side of the pre-clean room was eroded to a depth of 1 — 2 inches.

The paint is peeling on the walls in the pre-clean room. The areas in the corners of the room seem to be in the worst condition.

All manufacturing equipment viewed was in acceptable condition, of sanitary design, and was appropriately clean. A number of pieces of equipment had been transferred to this location from the Blakely facility. No poorly constructed on inadequately designed pieces of equipment were observed. All equipment observed was permanently installed (bolted to floor or a platform), and appropriately sealed with caulking material. There were no poorly welded areas on the equipment observed. The weld on the chute at the peanut dump station in the pre-clean room was broken and in need of repair. No opened ended unused conduits or piping was observed.

All hoppers for peanut storage and transport are open top vessels. There were no areas of dirt of debris accumulated on overhead piping or conduits above any of this vessels noted during this audit. The conveyor above the #13 Roka de- stoner had been equipped with a cardboard top held on with duct tape to attempt to control product from blowing into the air and out of the conveyor. This conveyor had also been labeled as #1 using paper and duct tape. This was noted on everal different pieces of equipment in the facility. It was understood that these were used as equipment identification .narkers during installation and were being replaced with metal tags.

A delron guide rail cover above the bucket elevator near the raw nut dumper was damaged and coming loose from the equipment.

All sides of exterior of the building are surrounded by asphalt. The areas along the south and west sides of the plant had significant amounts of dirt and product debris piled up along the building. This creates a potential food source and harborage for insects and rodents and should e maintained clean.

All exterior doors were closed with marginal seals in place. There were a number of small gaps noted in the seals of a number of the doors. Each emergency exit door is maintained closed but not locked. Each door utilized for access by plant employees is equipped with a mechanical lock and is of a self-closing design.

There were hand-sanitizing stations located in the production areas of the facility. There are hand-washing facilities in the employee bathrooms. No employees were observed wearing gloves while working in this operation. No gloves were noted stored in non-designated locations.

Items requiring maintenance attention are noted during daily inspections of the equipment. There was no preventive maintenance database reviewed. The plant needs to consider developing a formal program which includes a complete list of items requiring maintenance, tasks by item, frequencies, issuance of work schedules, input of maintenance work performed, maintenance history, inventory of equipment, etc., and parts and control of stock in maintenance stores.

The plant restrooms and break room were clean and no issues were noted. Employees currently wear their own clothing and shoes to work in all areas of the facility. Employees wear hairnets and beardnets when in the plant. The plant needs to institute a written uniform policy where no employee street clothes would e exposed to product. The plant should also implement a plant designated shoe program with provisions for keeping the shoes in the plant. Employee clothing and shoes could potentially ring unwanted microorganisms, dirt, and debris into the operation. It was understood that most employee's leave their shoes are the plant when not in use. The plant should define guidelines requiring that all plant shoes be kept at the plant when not in use. No employees where observed carrying items that could become potential foreign material in pockets above the waist. As a visitor, I was required to wear a hairnet.

There are currently no written plant guidelines for traffic control from raw to further processed. These requirements .nould include traffic patterns, uniforms requirements (needs, changes, etc.), hairnet requirements, shoe requirements, fork truck controls, etc. It was understood that the operators typically work in one area.

The operator in the sizing room that was operating the filler was observed touching the product and then handling the exterior of the new boxes to be filled. The employee was touching product to help top of the box to attain the correct weight. This employee should wear clean gloves to touch product, or an appropriate tool should be designated for this operation.

The pre-clean room was of negative air pressure to the further processing areas.

All areas of the product handling areas of the plant were adequately lighted with lights that were shielded or contained shatterproof bulbs.

Two wire brushes were observed near the blanchers (34 B / 34 A) roaster and under the hoppers in the pack out room. Wire brushes can be an excellent source of metal foreign material in a process and should be eliminated.

No non-cleaning chemicals items observed in the plant. The plant does not have a policy for these types of items. All approved non-cleaning chemicals should be included in a written control program that lists the item, the usage point (and amount if appropriate), and the storage location when not in use. Compliance to this should be part of the on-going internal plant inspections. There were no non-cleaning chemicals observed in locations they did not belong.

There were no temporary repairs of tape, wires, strings, etc., observed, but tape was used in the operational areas as mentioned above. There should be minimal use of tape in the operating areas and when used, it should be controlled - dated of application, inspected regularly for condition, and a plan of action to eliminate its need. With the exception of 1 electrical transfer / control panel in the pre-clean on the south wall with parts stored on top of it, I did not observe any items being stored in or on locations they did not belong (electrical cabinets, control panels, etc.)

Wooden handled brooms and other cleaning tools were observed in the plant operating areas. Efforts need to be made to eliminate wood from the product processing areas.

The plant operators conduct daily inspections of equipment and areas prior to starting up, and throughout operations.

Plant supervisors and managers conduct monthly internal audits. The entire plant interior and exterior is audited each month. These audits cover GMPs, housekeeping, operations, and sanitation. Any concerns are documented and corrective actions are assigned. Follow up occurs during future audits.

The granulation or sizing room is a separate room located adjacent to the finished product warehouse and has plastic strip curtain doors. Product is granulated and packed into finished product packages in this area. The airflow in the room was positive to the warehouse. There was some peeling paint observed on the housing of the bucket elevator by the sifter in this room.

The plant is in the process of adding an oil roasting line. The roasting equipment observed is in one corner of the finished product warehouse and the bulk infeed dump station (is same room as and) is about 30 feet from the pack-off station for blanched or roasted nuts. This process will need to be reviewed very closely prior to any start up to be sure that raw nuts are isolated from further processed nuts — this includes air flow, traffic flow, etc.

The plant has no documented supplier approval program. There are very few raw materials and packaging materials used in this facility. The plant sources raw materials and packaging materials from supplier that have long-term relationships with PCA and the other operating facilities.

The plant water is sourced from a municipal system. Water is primary for sanitation in this plant. The water is test annually by the city of Plainview for compliance to national drinking water standards. No testing results were reviewed as part of this audit. No additional testing is conducted on this water.

There are no bulk liquid ingredients received or utilized at this facility.

ALLERGEN CONTROL

Complying

The plant has an allergen statement in place and recognizes peanuts as allergens. The allergen statement is a general overview of allergens and includes a list of the top 8 allergens. Only peanuts are processed in this facility.

PCA would be responsible to notify Nest16 if there are any potential changes to the allergen status.

BIO-SECURITY

Complying with Major Improvement Needed

The plant does have a brief general plant safety policy. The plant has not completed any formal assessment of the site for bio-security. A formal assessment should be completed of the site and appropriate action taken against concerns noted.

The plant is located in a rural agricultural area about 40 miles north of Lubbock, Texas.

The site is fenced one 3 sides with the front of the building not being fenced. The front of the building has one entry door. There is one main gate for entering the fenced shipping and receiving areas. An employee must manually open this gate. The gate was noted standing open during the audit. The plant indicated a truck had just entered the site and the supervisor was going to close the gate. The supervisor was noted closing gate a few minutes later.

There are no security camera systems monitoring any areas of the building or grounds.

Employees and visitors must enter the building through one front door. Once in the building, you must walk past the plant offices to gain access to the production areas.

To employee is issued any type of identification badge, and there are no electronic locks. All visitors are escorted while on site.

All plant access doors were closed and not locked during the audit. Truck drivers may enter the building near the shipping / receiving office and must stay in this area.

There are emergency exit doors to the outside of the plant. These doors were found to be closed and not locked during the audit. The doors are equipped with handles on the exterior side and are self-closing.

The plant has a seals program, and there are seal's utilized on all inbound and outbound loads of raw material or finished product. It was understood that the plant would reject any raw material received without an intact numbered seal that is matched to the shipping documentations.

A trailer inspection program is in place to document the conditions of each trailer and load of materials received, and empty trailers prior to loading for shipment. The incoming and outgoing forms contain sufficient information to insure trailers are being inspected adequately.

There are no liquid bulk ingredients or chemicals received or stored at this location.

HACCP (HAZARD ANALYSIS CRITICAL CONTROL POINT)

Complying with Major Improvement Needed

A documented HACCP plan (dated December 29, 2005) based on the plan for the Blakely, Georgia plant has been developed. The plan was developed by the operations manager, quality manager, and technical director. The HACCP plan included process flow charts, CCPs, and corrective action plans. It was understood that a HACCP plan review is completed whenever there is a change to existing equipment, or when new equipment is added to the existing process line. The plant maintains a revisions history and log to track all changes to the HACCP plan. All paperwork that contains a CCP check is reviewed by plant and quality supervision.

Management has limited training in HACCP, but understands the basic principles of food safety related hazards. It is recommended that someone in management attend a certified HACCP training course to better understand food safety hazards that potentially occur through the entire product process flow from raw peanuts to finished roasted peanuts. Once complete, the HACCP program can be further reviewed and risk re-assessed. Risk assessment includes safety hazards related to microbiological, physical, and chemical (includes allergens) hazards. Currently the food safety concerns are centered on the physical presence of raw peanuts being handled in the peanut roasting area (microbiological).

The HACCP plan needs to include the following: risk assessment of processes and materials, process flow charts, CCPs, corrective action plans, meeting notes from HACCP discussions that might provide rationale for decisions (plan history), documentation of the process validation steps for CCPs, calibrations requirements, and documented outcomes of HACCP reviews.

A foreign material protection plan includes the following: a plant glass and brittle plastics policy is maintained, destoning equipment, in line screens / sifters, magnets, metal detectors, visual inspection of equipment prior to start up, and visual inspection of process of the operating condition and equipment during production.

The plant has 1 CCP for product that might be produced for Nestlê:

CCP 1 — roaster conditions. The dry roaster is operated such that peanuts are roasted at >/= 300 F for ab6ut 25 minutes.

The metal detection check was verified during this audit with no concerns noted. The system viewed was verified using 2.0 stainless steel, 2.0 non-ferrous, and 1.5 ferrous standards.

Metal detector monitoring procedures are established and include action in case of deviation. The systems are checked at least one time per hour by the quality control technician. .

Comments / concerns related to HACCP and the current plant design / usage related to concerns for potential microbiological cross contamination with the raw and finished nuts. These items need to be reviewed by the plant / company HACCP authorities.

The storage, dumping, and cleaning of raw nuts takes place in the pre-clean room. This room has a negative air pressure to the other areas of the plant. The room has a doorway entering into the roasting room, but no door is installed. What check is in place to be sure air pressure is maintained?

All peanut pieces are moved through the processing equipment via open top conveyors and bucket conveyors. All storage bins and conveyors are designed without any tops. The concern is for potential foreign material to easily enter the product flow.

Employees wear their street clothes in all areas of the operation. At a minimum, a smock or outer garment should be provided by the plant to create a barrier between the employee clothes and the product being processed.

There are informal traffic patterns and practices for moving vehicles and plant personnel, but no documented plant guidelines. A formal written control plan for the movement of personnel and equipment for the prevention of raw / further processed product contamination needs to be developed. This should include requirements for work assignments and personnel movement, uniform control / changes, hair net usage / changes, glove requirement, cleaning requirements, footwear treatments, etc.

Raw and blanched peanuts are roasted and / or blanched on specific equipment that has been installed on a shared line. The roaster is used to transport peanuts to the blanchers when the plant is blanching, and the blanchers are by-passed when roasting. The conveyors after these are share pieces of equipment. No microbiological studies have been completed to show that no risk is present on these shared pieces of equipment.

No environmental sampling program is in place or has been completed to provide information on the potential microbiological risks or concerns in the further processing areas.

The plant is in the process of installing an oil roasting system in a corner of the finished product warehouse. The peanut dumping station for the oil roasting system is being installed in the corner of the roasting / blanching room about 30 feet from the pack-off station for roasted / blanched nuts. By design, blanched only raw nuts will have to be transported to, and then dumped, in the roasting / blanching room.

QMS (Quality Monitoring Scheme)

Complying

Although a program formally called "QMS" does not exist, procedures and policies, manufacturing parameters, qualitycesting targets with ranges, specifications, corrective actions, and product/customer specific requirements are in place.

Results from quality testing are recorded throughout production on designated paperwork. Quality testing is completed throughout processing by quality control and production operators. The quality technicians are responsible to calibrate all equipment utilized for quality testing on a daily basis. Production and quality employees and supervisors are continually monitoring the quality of products through visuals inspections.

Typically, routine product testing includes visual, odor, microbiological, and analytical before, during and after manufacturing. The results can be included on a Certificate of Analysis (COA) as requested by each customer. Testing of the products produced is based on customer requirements. Testing typically includes:

Analytical — color, salt content, granulation or particulate sizing, odor, flavor may be informally tested

Organoleptic - aroma, appearance, and occasionally, flavor may be informally tested

Microbiological — aerobic plate count, yeast, mold, e. coli, salmonella, and coliforms — completed by an outside microbiological laboratory. Aflatoxin results are included on the COA, but these testing results are transferred from the information provided by the incoming results from the sheller.

All tasks and specifications are defined and completed for each lot produced. Additional customer specific testing requirements can be discussed and added if determined necessary.

The factory employees and management personnel I talked too were well aware of the product specifications, HACCP CCPs, and quality testing parameters.

Information is provided by the shellers for the incoming raw, shelled nuts. The results are from USDA parameters and testing for peanut grading. For testing purposes, a 75,000-gram samples is drawn across about 200, 000 pound lots.

Slot screen sizing
Percent other types of kernels
Split or broken kernels
Damaged or unshelled kernels
Minor defects
Foreign material based on 8, 012.60 grams.
Moisture
Aflatoxin (typically by J. Leek & Associates)

PATHOGEN MONITORING OF THE PRODUCTION ENVIRONMENT

Not Complying

There is currently no environmental pathogen-monitoring plan. There has been no pathogen-monitoring plan completed to provide historical information to justify the discontinuance of an environmental monitoring program for the operating areas of the facility.

A plan needs to be developed and implemented. If needed, Nest16 can provide recommendations for an appropriate sampling plan.

FORMAL RELEASE / STATUS CONTROL SYSTEM

Complying with Major Improvement Needed

All product currently produced in the facility is subject to a release practice. If products are processed according to the designated parameters, including a review of the CCPs, and they meet the testing requirements, they are considered ready for shipping. There are no computer transactions or paperwork processed to let the shipping areas know that the product has been checked and is ready for release. There is no documented "formal" release system in place; however, practices appear to be in place to prevent any out of compliance materials from being shipped.

It is recommended that a formal release system be create with an appropriate procedures and a formal release checklist utilizing testing and monitoring that is currently performed. A finished product microbial test is a good test to use as a finished product release criteria.

It was understood that all finished product is tested for pathogens prior to distribution. A certificate of analysis (COA) is generated for every lot of product shipped.

A written procedure is in place for the holding of non-conforming goods. The procedure reviewed was dated December 29, 2005. Non-conforming product would be tagged with a hold tag and moved to a designated area of the warehouse. The QA Manager has product disposition authority, but in some cases, may discuss these matters with the plant manager and company president.

LOT TRACEABILITY, LOT IDENTIFICATION, CODING / RECALL & CRISIS MANAGEMENT (MOCK RECALL)

Complying with Major Improvement Needed

A recall, mock recall, and crisis management procedure are documented and readily available. The recall procedure (dated December 29, 200) was reviewed during this audit. The procedure lists necessary steps in the event of a product recall and includes 24-hour emergency contact information.

It was understood that the plant conducted a mock recall during 2005, but no documentation was completed. No documentation is equal "did not happen". This does not meet Nestlé requirements.

PCA needs to develop and implement a workable protocol for conducting mock recalls and then it on a regular basis. The requirement is to be able to accurately locate and account for any lot of raw material or primary packaging material used from receipt through usage and finished product and on to the transfer of ownership of the finished goods. To be in compliance this must be completed within 2 hours. Further, a program must be in place to perform mock recalls and traces yearly and to analyze the results of the tests.

Based on paperwork reviewed, I believe that products and ingredients can be traced forward to orders and backward to dicoming raw material.

The plant does not have a written rework procedure to describe how rework product (when and if used) should be handled and tracked during manufacturing finished product label is printed in house and contains the following information:

Product name
Item number
Lot number T6005
T - Texas,
6 - year
005 - Julian day of manufacturing
Manufacturing date 1/5/06 (month/day/year)
Net weight

INSTRUMENT CALIBRATION (FOR CCPS) / LABORATORIES AND TEST METHOD

Complying with Major Improvement Needed

There is a quality control laboratory with equipment utilized for analytical product testing. No microbiological testing is completed at this site. All laboratory equipment is calibrated on a daily basis by the quality control technician. Calibration logs maintained for each piece of equipment were reviewed during the audit and found to be complete through today's date.

Plant scales are calibrated on an annual basis by Buffalo Gap Scale Company. The scales were last inspected on August 11, 2006. All scales are verified on a daily basis by the quality control and production operators.

The time/temperature recording devices and the thermocouples for the roasting line should be on a minimum annual calibration verification program by the vendor. These devices were originally calibrated by the manufacturer and have been operating for about 9 months. A written program needs to be established to be sure these devices are inspected / alibrated at leas annually, or as needed.

The metal detection systems for the roasting / granulation lines should be on a minimum annual calibration verification program by the vendor. These devices were originally calibrated by the manufacturer and have been operating for about 9 months. A written program needs to be established to be sure these devices are inspected / calibrated at least annually, or as needed. The quality control technicians verify the operation of these units prior to start up each day and then on an hourly basis throughout operations.

The magnets for the roasting line should be inspected annually for pull strength. A written program needs to be established to be sure these devices are inspected / replaced annually, or as needed as indicated by test results.

KEY ISSUES

Training

Complying

Although training practices are in place, there is no overall documented written training plan, which summarizes the training programs and plant training requirements. A formal written training plan containing plant / company training requirements should be written.

It is recommended that the plant implement a process by which learning effectiveness is measured. This can be completed by use of short tests following each training session.

Documentation

Complying

The plant should create a written Change Management policy that defines steps to be followed for changes that might take place in manufacturing and documentation.

Pencils were being utilized in the quality control areas. The facility should put forth an effort to eliminate pencils and use blue or black pens in all areas.

GMPs — Housekeeping

Complying with Major Improvement Needed

There were small amounts of peanut pieces along the south wall and behind electrical panels in the pre-clean room.

The exterior areas on the south and west sides of the plant had large amount of dirt and product debris (skins) scattered in depths for about $^1/4$ inch to about 8 inches.

There is a remote building on the north side of the plant, which contains what appears to be excess equipment and items removed from the plant. There is a large amount of items stored in piles on the ground. This creates potential harborage areas for insects, rodents, and birds. The building on the southwest corner of the plant used to park the skins collection trailer has unacceptable amounts of product skins accumulated on the floor areas.

A number of brooms and shovels have wooden handles. Any tools with wooden handles in the manufacturing areas of the plant should be replaced with non-wooden handled items.

There was a designated perimeter painted white about 18 inches wide maintained around the warehouse areas. This perimeter was free and clear of product storage, equipment storage, and any other unwanted dirt or debris. Along the exterior southwest wall of the pre-clean room, the concrete at the floor / wall juncture is eroded to a depth of 1 to 2 inches. This area was collecting dirt and debris and is not readily cleanable.

GMPs — Sanitation

Complying

The plant has established basic cleaning procedures and instructions for the pieces of equipment in the operation. These procedures are developed only for the major tasks. The cleaning standard operating procedures (SOPs) need to be developed throughout the plant to address all wet and dry cleaning. SOPs should be written to outline each task, the cleaning frequency, who is responsible for cleaning, chemicals to be used, chemical concentrations, personal protective equipment, tools needed to complete the task, and anything other information the plant personnel might need for these tasks.

The Master Cleaning Schedule is very basic, and does not include a number of items in the plant such as walls, ceilings, dr vents, electrical panels, floor drains, etc. All exterior areas of the plant should be added to master cleaning schedules as poor conditions can lead to potential infestations issues. All of these items should also have procedures developed as described above.

GMPs - Pest Control

Not Complying

Each device is inspected by the PCO during the site visit. All results are documented on the service reports. The plant should work with the PCO to develop a sheet that documents pest activity in a manner that trends can easily be seen. The sheets should be able to easily indicate problem areas or areas of concerns.

The pest control logs for the past 10 months were reviewed with varying levels of rodent activity noted on every report. The activity was primarily noted on the exterior of the building, but there were also concerns in the interior areas of the building. The pest control reports indicate that the plant has an on-going concern with rodent activity occurring at varying levels. The number of devices originally utilized in the service program was doubled after about 5 months of service. The service reports reviewed also say, "seal all voids around doors to prevent pest entry", without noting for which door is a concern. The PCO has utilized a straight line out to indicate some of the devices are being inspected. Each and every device that is inspected should be marked on the log sheet with an individual mark.

During the audit of the exterior of the building, the following was observed:

1. A bait box on north side of building near ramp was missing the top. The rodenticide was on the ground about 2 feet from the stations. There was another bait station installed about 4 feet away from the damaged bait station.
2. The partition walls around the exterior compressor room on the south west corner of the building are constructed of 2 layers of metal with about 3 inches of space in-between the layers. The area inside of this wall was easy viewed (due to the way they had been cut off) contained about 8 to 10 inches of dirt, product debris (skins), and mice carcasses.
3. Mouse carcass lying near bait station #10.
4. 3 mice carcasses and burrows under the grating located near on the wall near the shipping doors.
5. 3 mice carcasses in varying stages of decay lying near bait station #11.
6. 4 mice carcasses in varying stages of decay lying near bait station #12.
7. > 14 mice carcasses in varying stages of decay lying near bait station #13.
8. 5 mice carcasses in varying stages of decay lying near bait station #14.
9. > 10 mice carcasses in varying stages of decay lying near bait station #15.
10. 1 mice carcass in varying stages of decay lying near bait station #18.
11. 3 mice carcasses and 1 rat carcass in varying stages of decay lying near bait station #20.
12. 5 mice carcasses and 1 rat carcass in varying stages of decay lying near bait station #21.
13. 1 mouse carcass in the foam insulation near the corner of the building (area near emergency exit door on the south wall for the pre-clean room).
14. Numerous burrows along area on south side of plant where asphalt ends and dirt begin.
15. A dead pigeon was lying on the ground near the peanut-receiving door.

16. 4 pigeons roosting on the iron support structure inside the skin collection building. The doors to this outside building where hanging open, as the trailer was not completely backed into the building. Based on the feces observed, and by building design, it appears as if bird activity is a problem (and a potential problem) for this building.
17. A lot rodenticide was scattered loosely on the ground on the south and southwest exterior of the building.

From my observations during the audit walk through and from the pest control program records, plant management needs to review and revise the current program to incorporate more Integrated Pest Management techniques. This plant has a serious on-going problem with rodents on the exterior portions of the building must be resolved. Although there were no observations of rodents or rodent activity in the interior of the plant noted during this audit, the levels of dead rodents observed, coupled with voids noted around some doorways, indicate there are potential concerns for the interior areas of the plants.

Overall, the current pest control program appears to be less than effective and is unacceptable.

GMPs - Other

Complying with Major Improvement Needed

There were no open holes observed in the walls or floors from previous installations, however there were several pipe penetrations through interior walls in the pre-clean room that had not yet been sealed around.

Some of the concrete flooring was cracked and broken. This was in particularly poor condition were previous existing walls had been removed. The concrete at the floor / wall juncture on the west side of the pre-clean room was eroded to a depth of 1– 2 inches.

The paint is peeling on the walls in the pre-clean room. The areas in the corners of the room seem to be in the worst condition.

The weld on the chute at the peanut dump station in the pre-clean room was broken and in need of repair.

All hoppers for peanut storage and transport are open top vessels. There were no areas of dirt of debris accumulated on overhead piping or conduits above any of this vessels noted during this audit.

The conveyor above the #13 Roka de-stoner had been equipped with a cardboard top held on with duct tape to attempt to control product from blowing into the air and out of the conveyor. This conveyor had also been labeled as #1 using paper and duct tape. This was noted on several different pieces of equipment in the facility.

A delron guide rail cover above the bucket elevator near the raw nut dumper was damaged and coming loose from the equipment.

All sides of exterior of the building are surrounded by asphalt. The areas along the south and west sides of the plant had significant amounts of dirt and product debris piled up along the building. This creates a potential food source and harborage for insects and rodents and should e maintained clean.

All exterior doors were closed with marginal seals in place. There were a number of small gaps noted in the seals of a number of the doors. Each emergency exit door is maintained closed but not locked. Each door utilized for access by plant employees is equipped with a mechanical lock and is of a self-closing design.

Employees currently wear their own clothing and shoes to work in all areas of the facility. Employees wear hairnets and beardnets when in the plant. The plant needs to institute a written uniform policy where no employee street clothes would e exposed to product. The plant should also implement a plant designated shoe program with provisions for keeping the shoes in the plant. Employee clothing and shoes could potentially ring unwanted microorganisms, dirt, and debris into the operation. It was understood that most employee's leave their shoes are the plant when not in use. The plant should define guidelines requiring that all plant shoes be kept at the plant when not in use.

There are currently no written plant guidelines for traffic control from raw to further processed. These requirements should include traffic patterns, uniforms requirements (needs, changes, etc.), hairnet requirements, shoe requirements, fork truck controls, etc. It was understood that the operators typically work in one area.

The operator in the sizing room that was operating the filler was observed touching the product and then handling the exterior of the new boxes to be filled. The employee was touching product to help top of the box to attain the correct weight. This employee should wear clean gloves to touch product, or an appropriate tool should be designated for this operation.

Two wire brushes were observed near the blanchers (34 B / 34 A) roaster and under the hoppers in the pack out room. Wire brushes can be an excellent source of metal foreign material in a process and should be eliminated.

No non-cleaning chemicals items observed in the plant. The plant does not have a policy for these types of items. All approved non-cleaning chemicals should be included in a written control program that lists the item, the usage point (and amount if appropriate), and the storage location when not in use.

With the exception of 1 electrical transfer / control panel in the pre-clean on the south wall with parts stored on top of it, I did not observe any items being stored in or on locations they did not belong (electrical cabinets, control panels, etc.)

Wooden handled brooms and other cleaning tools were observed in the plant operating areas. Efforts need to be made to (iminate wood from the product processing areas.

The granulation or sizing room is a separate room located adjacent to the finished product warehouse and has plastic strip curtain doors. There was some peeling paint observed on the housing of the bucket elevator by the sifter in this room.

The plant is in the process of adding an oil roasting line. The roasting equipment observed is in one corner of the finished product warehouse and the bulk infeed dump station (is same room as and) is about 30 feet from the pack-off station for blanched or roasted nuts. This process will need to be reviewed very closely prior to any start up to be sure that raw nuts are isolated from further processed nuts — this includes air flow, traffic flow, etc.

The plant has no documented supplier approval program. There are very few raw materials and packaging materials used in this facility. The plant sources raw materials and packaging materials from supplier that have long-term relationships with PCA and the other operating facilities.

Bio-Security

Complying with Major Improvement Needed

The plant does have a brief general plant safety policy. The plant has not completed any formal assessment of the site for bio-security. A formal assessment should be completed of the site and appropriate action taken against concerns noted.

No employee is issued any type of identification badge, and there are no electronic locks.

AACCP (Hazard Analysis Critical Control Point)

Complying with Major Improvement Needed

Management has limited training in HACCP, but understands the basic principles of food safety related hazards. It is recommended that someone in management attend a certified HACCP training course to better understand food safety hazards that potentially occur through the entire product process flow from raw peanuts to finished roasted peanuts. Once complete, the HACCP program can be further reviewed and risk re-assessed. Risk assessment includes safety hazards related to microbiological, physical, and chemical (includes allergens) hazards. Currently the food safety concerns are centered on the physical presence of raw peanuts being handled in the peanut roasting area (microbiological).

Comments / concerns related to HACCP and the current plant design / usage related to concerns for potential microbiological cross contamination with the raw and finished nuts. These items need to be reviewed by the plant / company HACCP authorities.

The storage, dumping, and cleaning of raw nuts takes place in the pre-clean room. This room has a negative air pressure to the other areas of the plant. The room has a doorway entering into the roasting room, but no door is installed. What check is in place to be sure air pressure is maintained?

All peanut pieces are moved through the processing equipment via open top conveyors and bucket conveyors. All storage bins and conveyors are designed without any tops. The concern is for potential foreign material to easily enter the product flow.

Employees wear their street clothes in all areas of the operation. At a minimum, a smock or outer garment should be provided by the plant to create a barrier between the employee clothes and the product being processed.

There are informal traffic patterns and practices for moving vehicles and plant personnel, but no documented plant guidelines. A formal written control plan for the movement of personnel and equipment for the prevention of raw / further processed product contamination needs to be developed. This should include requirements for work assignments and personnel movement, uniform control / changes, hair net usage / changes, glove requirement, cleaning requirements, footwear treatments, etc.

Raw and blanched peanuts are roasted and / or blanched on specific equipment that has been installed on a shared line. The roaster is used to transport peanuts to the blanchers when the plant is blanching, and the blanchers are by-passed when roasting. The conveyors after these are share pieces of equipment. No microbiological studies have been completed to show that no risk is present on these shared pieces of equipment.

No environmental sampling program is in place or has been completed to provide information on the potential microbiological risks or concerns in the further processing areas.

The plant is in the process of installing an oil roasting system in a corner of the finished product warehouse. The peanut dumping station for the oil roasting system is being installed in the corner of the roasting / blanching room about 30 feet from the pack-off station for roasted / blanched nuts. By design, blanched only raw nuts will have to be transported to, and then dumped, in the roasting / blanching room.

Pathogen Monitoring of the Production Environment

Not Complying

There is currently no environmental pathogen-monitoring plan. There has been no pathogen-monitoring plan completed to provide historical information to justify the discontinuance of an environmental monitoring program for the operating areas of the facility.

A plan needs to be developed and implemented. If needed, Nestlê can provide recommendations for an appropriate sampling plan.

Formal Release / Status Control System

Complying with Major Improvement Needed

There is no documented "formal" release system in place; however, practices appear to be in place to prevent any out of compliance materials from being shipped.

It is recommended that a formal release system be create with an appropriate procedures and a formal release checklist testing and monitoring that is currently performed. A finished product microbial test is a good test to use as a finished product release criteria.

Lot Traceability, Lot Identification, Coding I Recall & Crisis Management (Mock Recall)

Complying with Major Improvement Needed

It was understood that the plant conducted a mock recall during 2005, but no documentation was completed. No documentation is equal "did not happen". This does not meet Nestlé requirements.

PCA needs to develop and implement a workable protocol for conducting mock recalls and then it on a regular basis. The requirement is to be able to accurately locate and account for any lot of raw material or primary packaging material used from receipt through usage and finished product and on to the transfer of ownership of the finished goods. To be in compliance this must be completed within 2 hours. Further, a program must be in place to perform mock recalls and traces yearly and to analyze the results of the tests.

Instrument Calibration (for CCPs) / Laboratories and Test Method

Complying with Major Improvement Needed

The time/temperature recording devices and the thermocouples for the roasting line should be on a minimum annual calibration verification program by the vendor. These devices were originally calibrated by the manufacturer and have been operating for about 9 months. A written program needs to be established to be sure these devices are inspected / calibrated at leas annually, or as needed.

The metal detection systems for the roasting / granulation lines should be on a minimum annual calibration verification rogram by the vendor. These devices were originally calibrated by the manufacturer and have been operating for about months. A written program needs to be established to be sure these devices are inspected / calibrated at least annually, or as needed. The quality control technicians verify the operation of these units prior to start up each day and then on an hourly basis throughout operations.

The magnets for the roasting line should be inspected annually for pull strength. A written program needs to be ;tablished to be sure these devices are inspected / replaced annually, or as needed as indicated by test results.

In: The Salmonella Outbreak in Peanut Products: The FDA ... ISBN: 978-1-60741-950-1
Editor: Benjamin K. Glynn

Chapter 25

SALMONELLA & INDUSTRY ROLE IN PROTECTION HEARING- AIB 2008 AUDIT

AIB International

RATING

A food safety audit was conducted at this facility on March 27, 2008.

The writer was accompanied throughout the audit by Mr. Danny Kilgorei' - Operations Manager, and Ms. Annie Bristow, Janitorial and Sanitation Director.

Excellent cooperation was received by the writer, and on some occasions, the items were immediately corrected.

At the conclusion of the audit, a meeting was held to discuss the observations, recommendationi, and rating The meeting was held with Mr. Danny Kilgore; Operations Manager.

Based on the observations made, theinformation obtained, and the-criteria set forth in *the AIB Consolidated Standards for Food Safety;* the overall food safety level of this facility was considered to be:

SUPERIOR (910)

The "serious" or "unsatisfactory" items are shaded, boxed, and bolded in the text of the report. Refer to thedefinitioni in the AIR Consolidated Standards:

The "improvement needed" items are designated in bold type and require prompt attention.

The AIB International statesthat the itport as given herein is to be construed as its findings and recommendations as of the date of this report. The AIS International accepts no responsibiliiy and does not assume any responsibility for the food safety program *in effect* with (customer). That Bother AIB International is only making report of the food safety conditions of (customer) as of the date-of • this report and assumes no responsibility or liability as to whether (customer) carries out the recommendations as contained in this report or does not carry out the recommendations as contained in this report.

Rating Analysis

DATE OF AUDIT:	March 27, 2008
TYPE OF AUDIT:	Announced
OVERALL RATING:	SUPERIOR
ADEQUACY OF FOOD SAFETY PROGRAM	175
PEST CONTROL	195
OPERATIONAL METHODS AND PERSONNEL PRACTICES	175
MAINTENANCE FOR FOOD SAFETY	175
CLEANING PRACTICES	190
TOTAL:.	910

Incidence Frequency Report (IFR)

	AI	PC	OP	MS	CP	*TM	UN	SER
PLANT OVERVIEW	3	2		0	1	7	0	0
EXTERIOR AND ROOF	0	0	0	1	0	1	0'	0
SUPPORT AREAS	0.	0	0	I -	0	1	0	0
MAINTENANCE AREAS	0	0	1	0	0	1	0	0
WAREHOUSE	0	0	0	0	0	0	0	0
PEANUT BUTTER AND PASTE OPERATIONS	0	0	1	2	2	5	0	0
TOTAL ITEMS BY CATEGORY	3	2	3	4	3		0ˉ	0

*TBA = TOTAL ITEMS BY AREA
AP = Adequacy of Food Safely Program
PC = Pcst Control
OP = Operational Methods and Personnel Practices
MS = Maintenance for Food Safety CP = Cleaning Practices
UN = Unsatisfactory
SER = Serious

Factual Observations and Specific Recommendations

Plant Overview

1. COM A current organizational chart dated January 12, 2008, was maintained.

The responsibility and authority for ensuring food safety and security, and the facility's compliance with federal, state, governmental, and/or any other' appropriate regulatory laws or guidelines were clearly assigned to the Operations Manager. This responsible person remains up to date on regulatory issues and has obtained the required regulatory food security registration dated 11/0/03.

2. COM A Food Safety Manual had been developed. This manual included,work instructions and/or job descriptions outlining the specific responsibilities of each department manager and employees, a Quality Policy signed by the Company President with a revision date of January 28, 2006, and written pcilicies for the programs listedin the *AIB Consolidated Standards for Food Softy.*

3. AP This facility had established a multidisciplinary food safety committee to conduct monthly inspections of theentire plant Inspection* were generally performed by the Operations'Manager and/or Janitorial/Sanitation Director. Documentation of the monthly Inspections included identified deficiencies, specific 111111VIDIVOI, and 'actual iccomplishmeuts. Inspections reviewed included January, 2008, February, 2008, and March, 2008. Follow-up inspections were done to ensure that the items were corrected. In addition, systenss and procedures critical to product safety and quality were audited to ensure they were in place, eppropriate, and complied with. This audit was-performed by the'Quality Assurance Manager and Operations Manger annually, most recently on January 12, 2008, by the Operations Manager. Continued attention to kein•that had the potential to impact` product zones was recommended. hems such as the paste room hoist maintenance, dealing and sealing gapi in vertical support beams and open ingredient containerwin the peanut butter mixing area. (IMPROVEMENT NEEDED)

4. COM The facility appeared to maintain an adequate budget and support to maintain the proper and timely acquisition of appropriate tools, materials, equipment, monitoring devices, chemicals, and pest control materials:

5. AP A Master Cleaning Schedule (MCS) and a daily housekeeping schedule were developed as a formalized, written plan and implemented in this facility. This MCS specified frequency and responsibility. Postcleaning evaluations were conducted. The schedules were documented as current, and the conditions observed in the plant supported the documentation. The schedule included the outside grounds, buildings, drains, and equipment. The schedule was reviewed periodically to insure that it was still applicable. Continued emphasis on cleaning the edges around the peanut butter pour-up stations and the floor/wall junctions and gaps in the paste room were needed.

6. COM Detailed, written cleaning procedures were developed and *on* file for all clasping tasks in the facility. These procedures included the chemicals, concentrations, tools, and disassembly instructions for equipment at the

level needed to facilitate the appropriate sanitation maintenance of the processing and packaging equipment, building areas, and outside grounds. Specific cleaning procedures were developed to prevent cross-contamination amid allergen and non-allergen-containing products.

7. COM Incoming goods and ingredients received into the facility west inspected according to established written procedures. The incoming goOds were checked for damage, cleanliness, and pest activity. The receiving records included date of receipt, carrier, lot number, amount, seal numbers (whets applicable), and product and vehicle conditions. Raw materials that contain allergens or are susceptible to raycotoxinsi autolysis &oils temperature abuse, or pathogenic microorganisms were segregated and covered by a separate written procedure with appropriate documentation.

8. COM Bulk deliveries of liquid materials included a visual inspection both before and after unloading. Verification was conducted that hatch and hoie seals matched' those listed on the bill of lading to ensure load integrity in transit. The findings were documented.

9. COM Appropriate specifications were on file for the raw materials, packaging terials, finished products, and intemsediate/semiprocessed products. These specifications were detailed to ensure compliance with relevant food safety and legislative requirements. These specifications were periodically reviewed and formally agreed upon with relevant parties.

10. COM Certificates of analysis and/or supplier guarantees for raw materials, od packaging, and finished products were maintained on file.

11. COM A Hazard Analysis Critical Control Point (HACCP) program had been eloped and "implemented for all processes and process lines. The progrram included the following components: Description of the products manufactured and hazards inherent to them, determined through risk assessment; Identification of critical control points (CCP) and criticatlimits; Procedures to control the CCPs; Deteiintitation of the monitoring frequency for the CCPs and destination of the person(s) responsible for testing; Established and dricumented deviation procedures; Written verification program, with proper documentation; Documentation of procedures, records of conformance, and corrective actions: This facility had evaluated the processes and procedures and determined that no critical control points were present in the operation. The designated monitoring control points (MCPs) were specified and described. The most recent program reassessment bad been performed by the Operations Manager on January 12, 2008.

12. COM The company had established written employee and Good Manufacturing Practices (GMPs) policies. Specific written procedures were on file for providing food safety training to all personnel, including temporary personnel and contractors. Employees alsd attended monthly food safety meetings that reviewed different aspects of food safety and GMPs. Records of training completion for new employees and annual refresher training documentation were nsaintained for all personnel. The

most recent employee meeting was held on 03/05/08. Items covered included AIB, GMP, hand sanitation, 10114 and clean-up. The annual employee training was held in January and February, 2008.

13. COM A written program for evaluating consumer complaint's was established at this location. This program 'included the rapid dissemination of complaint information to aUdepartments responsible for implementing.the food safety program. Complaint information was used, whereappropriat% to avoidrecurrenee and irnpliment ongoing improvements to product Safety, legality, and quality Actions appropriate to the seriousness and frequency of the probleins identified. appeared to be carried out promptly and effectively.

14. COM A written recall program was on file. All finished products wcie coded. Product traceability was accomplished through the recording of ray, material lot numbers on production records, and included source identification for work in progress and rework Distribution records were maintained to identify the initial point of distribution to facilitate segregation and recall of specific lots. The recall program was tested every six months with appropriate documentation maintained on file.

* The most recent mock recall was done on January 1'5, 2008. The incoming peanut lot number tracked was 14675 received on October 18, 2007, from `a known supplier. The peanut lot number was used in a number of manufactured products, manufacturing codes for 7 items were provided. The mock recall was completed in two hours and 15 minutes with 100 % effectiveness documented.'

15. COM Written procedures were in place to control nonconforming product, including work in progress, finished product, and returned goods. Corrective actions equal to the seriousness of the risk appeared to be taken. Records were kept of the corrective actions and disposition of the product The disposition records account for the total quantity of the'nonconforrning material produced.

16. COM A written policy on how to handle regulatory and third party inspections was on file. These procedures included Ulf person(s) delegated to accompany all inspectors and company policies regarding photographs, records, and samples. The most recent regulatory inspection was done by the Georgia Department of Agriculture, Consumer Protection Division, on December 14, 2007. No violations were noted.

17. COM A written program to evaluite and select suppliers of goods and services that affect product quality and food safety had been implemented. An approved list of these suppliers was maintained. An approved list of these Suppliers dated December 29, 2005, was maintained.

18. AP A written policy stating that no glass or brittle plastics were to be used in the facility, except where absolutely necessary, was in place. Included in the` policy was a prod on how to handle any glass breakage in the facility. A list of all essential glass had been developed and was audited on a routine frequency to ensure that any accidental breakage was found and addressed. The most recent audit was done on March 1, 2008. One

deficiency was observed during this audit. Additional attention to cracked light covers was 'recommended.

19. COM A found preventive maintenance program and work order system was in use to prioritize the elements of identified structural, equipment, or utensil maintenance problems that could cause food adulteration. The program listed the equipment and frequency of the work required to keep the equipment and facility well maintained and in good order. A program to ensure that the safety and legality of product were not jeopardized during maintenance operations was iniptemented at this facility.

20. COM This operation had established a formalized program for the control of bacteria, yeast, and mold as required. Records of laboratory analysis and/or environmental sampling were maintained. Environmental samples were sent to an approved, outside laboratory for testing. Finished product testing was determined by customer requirements and could include total plate count, conforms, E. coli, Salmonella, and Staphylococcus aureus. AU microbiological testing would be performed by an approved, outside laboratory. The on-site laboratory was maintained in such a manner as not to jeopardize the safety of product.

21. COM A formalized pest control program was established with written procedures' outlining the requirements of the program to reduce the potential for pniduct contamination from pest activity or use of materials and/or procedures designed to control pest activity.

22. COM Facility management contracted the McCall Services, Inc., Company to provide weekly pest control services for the exterior of the facility and the interior rodent, control program. Also, McCall Services, Inc., provided Weekly service for the interior insect light traps. A copy of the service agreement that included materials to be used, methods, and precautions was maintained on file. Copies of the current Georgia State Department of Agriculture license with an expiration dale of 06/30/09, liability insurance with expiration date of 08/01/08, and current applicator's license with an expiration date of 06/30/09 were maintained on file. In addition, Adams Pest Control was contracted to perform weekly interior crack and crevice pesticide applications in the facility and offices. Copies of the GeOrgia State Department of Agriculture license with an expiration date of 06/30/09, liability insurance with expiration date of 03/01/09, and current applicator's license with an expiration date of 06/30/09.

23. COM Material Safety Data Sheets (MSDS) and sample labels were maintained on file for all pesticides applied and/or stored on the premises.

24. COM A service report was left after each visit by the outside pest control service. These records included the treatments and tasks carried out, documentation of the checks and fmdings for the pest monitoring devices, descriptions of the current levels of pest activity, and recommendations for actions needed to correct conditions allowing a potential for pest activity. The most recent interior service date was

March 25, 2008, the most recent exterior service date was March 26, 2008.

25. COM Documentation of all pesticides applied on the premises, including rodenticides, included materials applied, target organism, amount applied, specific area where pesticide was applied, method of application; rate of application or dosage, date and time treated, and applicator's signature. This documentation indicated that the applications were made in accordance with the label directions. A pesticide list was provided. Pesticides used since the previous audit included Generation mini blocks, EPA registration number 7173-218 and Niban Granular Bait, # 64405-2. Entech Fog 5, # 40391-3, was used in the automatic fogging system on-site when needed. This system was operated by facility personnel. The Adams Pest Control pesticide being used for crack and crevice treatment was Bifen la, EPA registration # 53883-118.

26. COM Schematics depicting the locations of the interior and exterior pest control devices, including 60 mechanical Tin Cat rodent traps, four insect light traps, and 28 bait stations, were maintained on file and appeared current

27. PC Mechanical mousetraps were installed to monitor for rodent activity inside thee facility. These traps were properly positioned along walls and beside doors to the outside. The traps were inspected on a weekly basis, and a record was maintained of service and cleaning of 'each rodent control devicevA rodent activity log used to record captures and help direct any necessary corrective actions. The traps randomly examined appeared properly maintained. During the interior inspection, it was noted that several Tin Cats were found to be moved out of position. Employees should be reminded to replace a trap when it is moved due to cleaning or maintenance in order to maintain an effective rodent control program,

28. COM Bait stations for rodent control were installed around the exterior perimeter of the facility at appropriate intervals. These stations were tamper resistant, properly, ' positioned, anchored in place, locked, and properly labeled in compliance with regulatory requirements. All stations were serviced at least monthly. Fresh bait had been supplied MI= stations randomly examined. The service and results of the checks were documented on plastic punch cards inside each trap and on the pesticide usage sheets provided.

29. PC Electronic flying inliect light traps (1LTs) wire used in the facility to aid in monitoring insect activity. These traps were more than ten feet (three meters) from exposed product The traps were scheduled for weekly cleaning in the˙ summer and monthly cleaning in the winter. A record of the Service and cleaning of each ILT was maintained, and the activity levels documented. The light tubes were replaced annually and supporting documentation was maintained. The insect light trap located inside the caged ingredient storage room had ont Tight not working and

a glue board with many insects on it. The light bulb should be replaced and a new glue board should be installed.

30. COM Pheroinenz lures or traps were not currently in use in this facility.

31. COM All pesticides and application equipment used as pail of the on-site automatic fogging system were stored in a locked and ventilated room identified with appropriate signage. Materials to control spills or leakage were, provided in the storage enclosure. AU other pesticides and application equipment provided by the contract PCOs. No deviations were noted during the facility inspection.

32. COM No evidence of rodent or bird activity was noted in or around the facility.

33. OP. Eighteen-inch perimeters were generally maintained in all storage areas to provide cleaning and inspection access. Adequate space for cleaning was maintained betwetn rows of stored products. However, several cardboard boxes were stored on the perimeter in the UPS shipping comer and several buckets and containers on the perimeter inside the chemical storage cage. Items stored on the perimeter in the UPS shipping corner and the chemical cage should be elevated to allow inspection and cleaning

34. COM All incoming ingredients and packaging materials were dated on receipt to ease 'first-in, first-out stock rotation. A formal program was in place to monitor' and repelled= raw materials susceptible to stored product pest activity that were in storage for more than four weeks. Ingredients noted included stabilizer, flour salt, and molasses powder.

35. COM Materials in storage were adequately segregated to prevent contamination. Segregated storage•was provided for allergen containing ingredients, packaging materials, Research and Development items, cleaning and maintenance chemicals, nonconforming stock, and nonproduct related materials, such as parts and equipment.

36. COM Metal detection equipment was provided on each product line. The metal detectors were checked regularly throughout the shift using the relevant test pieces for 2.0 mm ferrous, 2.0 mm nonferrous, and 2.0 mm 316 stainless steel. The detectors employed &elite of both an alarm and a positive reject mechanism. Rejected material was diverted into a secured container or was removed from the line. Documentation of the checks was maintained. The detectors were checked duiing the sin-Vey and found properly to detect and reject thi provided testpieces. It was noted that the case metal detectors did not reject product but used a belt stop as the rejection method. This was due to the size of the container and the loose product involved. The peanut butter metal detector was a flow-thru unit and rejected into a container.

37. COM Procedures for corrective actions to respond to any failure of the metal detectors were on file. These included training, isolation, quarantining, and rcinspection of all food produced since the last aceeptable test of the metal detector.

38. COM Company policy required that all employees' cuts and grazes on exposed skin be covered by a company-issued metal detectable metal strip bandage. These bandages were tested on a predetermined frequency through a metal detector and supporting documentation was maintained.

39. COM All outside receiving lines or caps for bulk liquid ingredients were locked and identified. The liquid nitrogen tank and receiving line were located inside a locked fence enclosure.

40. COM Accessible and cleanable in-line receiving strainers had been provided for the bulk liquid ingredients. The strainer was examined on a per load basis, and documentation was maintained. The receiving strainer was checked during the survey and found clean and in good condition.

41. COM Adequate band washing and sanitizing stations were located at appropriate locations and used properly by the employees. "Wash Hands" signs were displayed in the rest rooms, hmthroom, and by sinks and 'entryways to production areas.

42. COM The washrooms and locker rooms were maintained in an acceptable Sanitary condition. The kickers were inspected monthly as a sanitary control, and no open food or drink was allowed.

43. COM A formal allergen program dated,January 18, 2005, and reviewed on January 12, 2008, was in place that included written policies and procedures. Effective measures were undertaken to prevent cross contamination amid incompatible. materials.

44. COM All shipping` vehicleswere inspected before loading for cleanliness and structural defects that could jeopardize product integrity, and documentation was maintained. Security seals were provided on and docuMented for all outbound vehicles.

45. COM Employees °Waved in the facility were wearing adequate hair and beard restraints. Their clothing and uniforms were clean and well maintained. No evidence of loose or unsecured jewelry was noted.

46. COM No evidence of eating, drinking, or smoking in unauthorized areas was observed. No smoking was allowed except on thoexterior of the facility.

47. COM All personal property was stored in appropriate loCations defined by company policy.

48. COM Some measures were undertaken to maintain site security. Site securitystrategies included fencing, controlled gate access al night, parking outside the fenced area, locked doors at night, employee entrance bad keypad entry, interior and exterior surveillance cameras, truck seals, employee screening, and awareness and traiiing programs.

49. COM The exterior grounds were adequately maintained to prevent pest harborage. Waste collection containers were located approximately 100 feet behind the facility and spillage was kept to a minimum.

50. COM Fixtures, ducts, and pipes were generally properly installed and maintained to prevent contamination from leaks, condensation, or insulating material.

51. COM Adequate ventilation was provided in the facility. Filters were in place in air make up units. Fans were maintained and operated in a manner to avoid product contamination.

52. COM A calibration program was in place for all regulating and recording controls. This was included as part of the facility Standard Operating Procedures. Accurate Scale Compatiy, alsorthe Georgia Department of Agriculture, Scales and Measures Division, tested the facility scales. The toaster companies, Proctor, AeroGlide, and Pittman oil masters wereused to standardize the roisteer control systems. Temperatures were monitored internally to assure proper temperature controL

53. COM Compressed air used in processing was properly filtered, and a program was in place to inspect and replace traps and/or filters.

54. COM Only food grade lubricants were used on food processing machines. These lubricants were fully segregated in a designated location, the maintenance shop.

55. COM Potable water was supplied from an appropriate source, the Blakely City Water System. A program was in place to monitor water quality. The facility had a report from the city based on the Clean Water Act requirements.

56. COM Devices were installed and maintained where appropriate¯to prevent backflow and/or back siphonage, While the facility did not have in-line back flow prevention devices, anti-siphon divices were observed on faucets located around and inside the facility.

57. COM All fluorescent light tubes,essential glass, and brittle plastic in the facility appeared to be protected from accidental breakage, or were accounted for in the Glass and Brittle PlasticS Management Program.

58. COM The floors, walls, and ceilings throughout the plant were generally of sound construction and well maintained. No roof leakage was evident.

59. COM An ongoing housekeeping program was in place throughout the hours of operation so that operational debris was kept to a minimum.

60. CP Adequate cleaning equipment and tools were available and stored away from the production areas. During the facility inspection, several wooden-handled utensils were observed, such as scrapers and sweepers. It was recommended that no wooden-handled utensils be used in food production areas due to the possibility of splintering or breakage.

61. COM The equipment was cleaned according to the MCS to prevent the development of microorganisms, insects, or foreign material.

62. COM Food contact cleaning surfaces and utensils were cleaned often enough to remove food residue`and maintain a good cosmetic appearance.

63. COM Only cleaning compounds and sanitizers that are authorized for use on food contact surfaces were used for cleaning. The chemical control program consisted of purchasing from approved vendors only. Materials rirchased were approved by the sanitation Director or maintenance manager prior to purchase. In addition, chemicals used for cleaning were kept in a locked cage inside the plant warehouse.

64. COM The. maintenance cleaning practices *were* found satisfactory. The maintenance debris, tools, and other items generated during maintenance activities were removed from the work area.

65. COM This facility had an automated Entech fogging system for fogging the interior of the plant. This system was operated inside a fenced, gated and locked enclosure inside the facility. It was noted that the plant used a pre-operational inspection procedure that included additional cleaning when noted on the inspection checklist. Thi pre-operational inspector would be notified when fogging had occurred and would require cleaning of product zones prior to releasing the equipment for operation. This general program was documented for review.

Exterior and Roof

66. COM No issues were observed on the roof of the facility. All air intakes were properly. screened to prevent any pest access into the facility.

67. MS A break in the concrete block wall was observed next to dock door 5 on the north exterior wall of the facility. The break in the concrete block should be properly sealed to prevent any possible pest entry or harborage in the block wall.

68. COM The paved areas around the facility had been repaired since the previous audit. No issues with standing water or potholes were noted.

69. COM During the exterior inspection, it was noted that the dumpsters used for trash or garbage were ,located away from the building. The dumpsters were open, but all trash in the dumpsters was being secured inside tied plastic bags. This would prevent possible pest (bird) attraction to the dumpsters.

Support Areas

70. COM The employee break room and employee Pest rooms were inspected and found to be properly cleaned and maintained.

71. MS In the wash room, a broken plastic light shield was observed. It was note&that all fluorescent lights in the facility were shatter-resistant However, the broken plastic should be removed to prevent possible fragmentation into the wash room. This was not an open product area.

Maintenance Areas

72. OP Maintenance areas inspected during the auditwere found to be generally clean and maintained. Continued to attention to storing items so that perimeter inspections can be performed was recommended.

Warehouse

73. COM	In the warehouse caged area, the insect light trap had a bulb that was not working. Also the glue board had a number of insects trapped. The light bulb should be replaced and the glue board should be replaced to provide an effectiye insect monitoring program in this stcliage area
74. COM	The top of the break room was inspected and found to be generally clean and properly maintained.
75. COM	The general warehouse storage areas were inspected and found to be properly organized and well maintained. No spillage or torn ingredient containers were observed.

Peanut Butter and Paste Operations

76.OP	In the peanut butter mixing operation, several instances of open Ingredient containers were observed in the area of the mixer located on the roof of the peanut butter room. Ingredient containers should be closed or secured when not in use in order to prevent possible product contamination due to materials falling into the ingredients being used. (IMPROVEMENT NEEDED)
77. MS	In the peanut butter room, the plastic motor fan cover for the blender motor was broken and damaged.'Whlle the blender was covered, the plastic cover could fragment and should be replacal
78. COM	In the votitor room, the peanut butter transfer piping passageway had loosened and created a gap in the wall seal. In order to prevent any possibility of insect , harborage, the wall opening should be re-sealed.
79. CP	In the corner by the peanut butter peanut pour-up stations, product Residue accumulation was noted on the horizontal beams and in the corner'at the floor/wall junction. Several live sawtooth grain beetles were noted in the residue. This area should be thoroughly cleaned and monitored to prevent further buildup and possible insect development.
80. MS	In the paste room the hoist cable had a label located above the peanut hopper that was peeling and could fall into the, peanut hopper. The label was immediately removed. Attention should be paid to all items located above open zones. (IMPROVEMENT NEEDED)
81. CP	In the northeast corner of the paste room, a gap was noted between vertical roof support beams. This gap bad product residue accumulated in the small opening between the beams. A live sawtobth grain beetle was found in the residue. This gap should be thoroughly cleaned to remove' all product residue. In addition, it was recommended that the gap be sealed with concrete to remove the gap and provide a cleanable surface.

CHAPTER SOURCES

The following chapters have been previously published:

Chapter 1 - These remarks were delivered as Statement of Darlene M. Cowart, Ph.D., President, JLA, USA, before the Subcommittee on Oversight and Investigation, U.S. House of Representatives, Energy and Commerce Committee, dated February 11, 2009.

Chapter 2 – These remarks were delivered as Statement of Charles T. Deibel, President, Deibel Laboratories, before the Subcommittee on Oversight and Investigation, U.S. House of Representatives, Energy and Commerce Committee, dated February 11, 2009.

Chapter 3 – These remarks were delivered as Statement of Peter K. Hurley, before the Subcommittee on Oversight and Investigation, U.S. House of Representatives, Energy and Commerce Committee, dated February 11, 2009.

Chapter 4 – This is an edited, excerpted and augmented email sent by Stewart Parnell to Sammy Lightsey, dated October 6, 2008.

Chapter 5 – This is an edited, excerpted and augmented email sent by Stewart Parnell, dated January 19, 2008.

Chapter 6 – This is an edited, excerpted and augmented email sent by Stewart Parnell, dated January 12, 2008.

Chapter 7 - This is an edited, excerpted and augmented edition Letter sent by Michelle Pronto to Hon. Henry A. Waxman, Chairman, Committee of Energy and Commerce and Hon. Bart Stupak, Chairman, Subcommittee on Oversight and Investigations, U.S. House of Representatives, Energy and Commerce Committee, dated February 10, 2009.

Chapter 8 – These remarks were delivered as Statement of Rep. Henry A. Waxman, Chairman, Committee on Energy and Commerce, before the Subcommittee on Oversight and Investigation, U.S. House of Representatives, Energy and Commerce Committee, dated February 11, 2009.

Chapter 9 – This is an edited, excerpted and augmented Department of Health and Human Services, Food adn Drug Administration Inspection Report on Peanut Corp., dated January 9, 2008.

Chapter 10 - This is an edited, excerpted and augmented edition of a United States Congressional Research Service publication, Report Order Code RL34167, updated September 16, 2008.

Chapter 11 – These remarks were delivered as Statement of Caroline Smith DeWaal, Director of Food Safety, before the Senate Committee on Agriculture, Nutrition and Forestry, dated February 5, 2009.

Chapter 12 – These remarks were delivered as Statement of William K. Hubbard, Alliance for a Stronger FDA, before the Senate Committee on Agriculture, Nutrition and Forestry, dated February 5, 2009.

Chapter 13 – These remarks were delivered as Statement of Ali Khan, MD, MPH, Assistant Surgeon General and Deputy Director, National Center for Zoonotic, Vector-borne, and Enteric Diseases, Centers for Disease Control and Prevention (CDC), U.S. Department of Health and Human Services, before the Senate Committee on Agriculture, Nutrition and Forestry, dated February 5, 2009.

Chapter 14 – These remarks were delivered as Statement of Gabrielle Meunier, Mother of *Sabnomella* Typhimurmium victim, before the Senate Committee on Agriculture, Nutrition and Forestry, dated February 5, 2009.

Chapter 15 – These remarks were delivered as Statement of Stephen F. Sundlof, D.V.M., PH.D, Director, Center for Food Safety and Applied Nutrition, Food and Drug Administration, U.S. Department of Health and Human Services, before the Senate Committee on Agriculture, Nutrition and Forestry, dated February 5, 2009.

Chapter 16 - These remarks were delivered as Statement of Rep. Henry A. Waxman, Chairman, Committee of Energy, before the Subcommittee on Oversight and Investigations, U.S. House of Representatives, Energy and Commerce Committee, dated March 19, 2009.

Chapter 17 - These remarks were delivered as Statement of Rep. Bart Stupak, Chairman, before the Subcommittee on Oversight and Investigations, U.S. House of Representatives, Energy and Commerce Committee, dated March 19, 2009.

Chapter 18 - These images were part of a Food and Safety Audit of Peanut Corporation of America facilities in Georgia and Texas, presented before the Subcommittee on Oversight and Investigations, U.S. House of Representatives, Energy and Commerce Committee, dated March 19, 2009.

Chapter 19 - These remarks were delivered as Statement of J. Martin Kanan, President and CEO Kanan Enterprises, Inc., before the Subcommittee on Oversight and Investigations, U.S. House of Representatives, Energy and Commerce Committee, dated March 19, 2009.

Chapter 20 - These remarks were delivered as Statement of A.D. David Mackay, President and CEO, Kellog Company, before the Subcommittee on Oversight and Investigations, U.S. House of Representatives, Energy and Commerce Committee, dated March 19, 2009.

Chapter 21 - These remarks were delivered as Statement of Heather C. Isely, Executive Vice President, Vitamin Cottage Natural Food Markets, Inc. (Natural Grocers), before the Subcommittee on Oversight and Investigations, U.S. House of Representatives, Energy and Commerce Committee, dated March 19, 2009.

Chapter 22 – This is an edited, excerpted and augmented email sent by Sammy Lightsey to Pete Hatfield, dated December 31, 2008.

Chapter 23 – This is an edited, excerpted and augmented email sent by Tim Slawinski to Jennifer Tong, dated December 31, 2008.

Chapter 24 – This is an edited, excerpted and augmented NQS Level 1 - Food Safety Audit Report by Nestle North America of Peanut Corporation of America, dated January 5, 2006.

Chapter 25 – This is an edited, excerpted and augmented AIB Food Safety Audit Report by Eugene A. Hatfield, Food Safety Auditor, of Peanut Corporation of America, dated March 27, 2008.

Index

A

B

C

D

E

F

G

H

I

J

K

L

M

N

O

P

Q

R

S

T

U

V

W

Y